A Sailor's Advice on Life

CLEVELAND O. EASON

Copyright © 2019 Cleveland O. Eason
All rights reserved
Second Edition

First originally published by Page Publishing 2020

ISBN 979-8-9892364-0-4 (pbk)
ISBN 979-8-9892364-2-8 (digital)

Printed in the United States of America

Contents

Preface 5

1. Emotions: What's in Your Seabag? 7
2. Relationships: How Do You Manage Them? 23
3. Room 4: How Do You Obtain Joy? 54
4. Money: Steward or Squander? 62
5. The Race: Starting and Finishing Strong 80

Preface

I am dedicating this book to my family (nuclear and extended), who pointed me in the right direction, and provided me the initial calibration for my personal compass. My personal compass has allowed me to make the course corrections I have had to make during my life's journey. During my life, I enjoyed the privilege of travel first with the US Army during my father's twenty-year military career, followed by my own twenty-three-year career with the US Navy, and post military retirement travel opportunities. (I'm not done traveling!) Traveling has allowed me to experience different cultures and meet people from different walks of life. During my courses of travel, I have made numerous observations and believe my observations would be of value for anyone who desires to avoid some of life's common pitfalls. Despite our differences (gender, race, religion, economic status, etc.), there are common threads we all share.

I believe this book can help guide a person who is starting out, starting over or in need of a course correction to discover the way to true North. When all else fails, it helps to get back to basics! In order to breakout from the pack and finish your race strong, you need self-discipline, desire, and a vision guided by a moral conscience. When I left home to join the US Navy at the tender age of seventeen (four weeks after my high school graduation), I was unaware my observations and experiences were allowing me to compile the information for this book. My young adult observations of life were in a post-Vietnam, Cold War era US Navy gave me the false impression that working hard and playing harder were all that mattered in life. Fortunately for me during my time in the desert of pleasures, my initial compass heading set by my home environment and people of virtue I met along the way, guided me to the oasis of joy.

The experiences I had during my early separation phase of life revealed to me that there is great value in understanding the issues related to emotions, relationships, and money. I am writing this book as a pathway to help those who strive to avoid the snares that life has for those who are walking its precarious road. I personally do not believe the "School of Hard Knocks" is the most time efficient way to obtain life's pearls of wisdom (unless you are going to live forever and be totally immune to any of the consequences of your decisions… not!) We have too many generations of people who repeat the errors of their predecessors and are stuck in a seemingly endless cycle of frustration and/or poverty. If you are thirsting for insight, knowledge, and wisdom, then you are in the right place. If you question my motives for writing this book, then I challenge you to read on and discover a man baring his soul so that many more people can enjoy the peace that comes with being aware of yourself and those around you.

I kept this book short because I learned from a Navy admiral to be brief, be brilliant, and be gone, the three elements of a successful speech! Despite this book's brevity, it provides keen insight into the "why" we do what we do and some "lessons learned" for those who want to learn from others' experiences. It is also for those who desire to get ahead in life with fewer instances of two steps forward and one step back!

Chapter 1

Emotions
What's in Your Seabag?

You're probably wondering why this book is starting with a subject so many people avoid trying to understand? If you have not figured it out by now, you can't underestimate the power of your emotions and how your emotions can compel you to do the unthinkable. If you think you are on an island, then it's time to wake up and smell the coffee! We all are influenced by our emotions. It does not matter what part of the world you are from; We all go through four phases of life: Preparation (age 0–18?), Separation (18–28?), Independence (28–??), and Dependent (85–??).

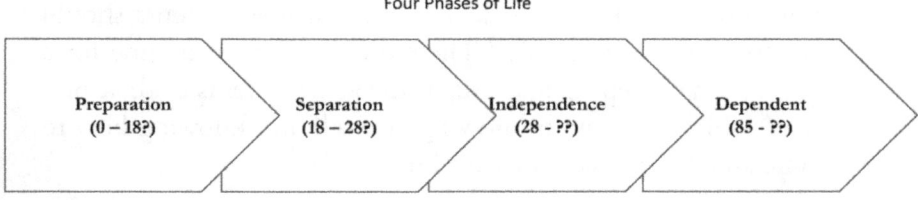

Figure 1 - 1

Some are slow to transition from one phase to the other and the ability to progress through the phases depends on what is in your emotional seabag. In the Navy, your "seabag" is where you put all the things you need to go on a six-month or longer voyage away from home. Sailors typically pack as much as they can in the seabag because once the ship leaves homeport, you can't go back and retrieve a forgotten item! Your emotional seabag is comprised of the experiences and relationships you had during the Preparation phase of life (which can vary in length and is based on the amount of parental/guardian interaction and/or social economic position.) Your ability to function during the Separation and Independence phases of life depends heavily upon what was put into your emotional seabag during the Preparation phase.

Understanding what is in your emotional seabag is important. To borrow a line from the Clint Eastwood movie, "Magnum Force" "A man's got to know his limitations," is why understanding what's in your emotional seabag is important. There is no one who has not been touched by the family experience. The thought of family can conjure up either feelings of joy and happiness, nightmares you prefer not to recall, or something in between. In fact, people who went through horrific times as children often spend the next ten to fifteen years (or even longer!) pursuing emotional happiness. Dysfunctional families affect all occupants of the global village. If you don't believe me, then just look at the crime statistics or other social ills and you will discover, that a lot of our society's problems are family issues. Governments can only address the symptoms (laws, law enforcement, criminal justice system, family court, etc.), and not the root of the problem, which is the deterioration of the family unit. Believe me, I am not advocating nor do I think that governments should get into the parenting business! Therefore, I believe it is time for a new generation to step-up and exceed the achievements of their predecessors, which starts with knowing yourself and knowing how to overcome and compensate for your limitations.

The Five "Relationship Needs" Accounts

Most people in this day and age have heard of the Maslow hierarchy of needs triangle.[1] This has been accepted as model for

---

[1] https://www.simplypsychology.org/maslow.html

human behavior and has had several updates since its initial inception, and for some, it seems to answer to "why people do what they do" question.

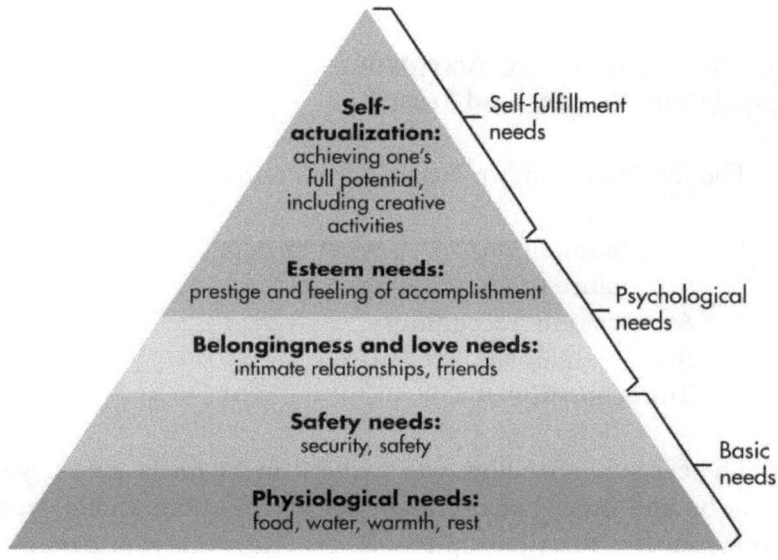

Figure 1 - 2
https://www.simplypsychology.org/maslow.html

There is validity in Maslow's needs model, and after many discussions with people from a myriad of backgrounds (economic, gender, racial, religious, etc.), I have discovered most relationships fail or are imbalanced when they lack sufficient levels of what I have identified as the "five relationship needs." The presence of love, acceptance, appreciation, respect, and trust are what motivate people to satisfy those needs with activities inside or outside of the relationship, or with or without external stimulates, such as alcohol, drugs, or other compulsive behavior. Caution—one relationship can't supply all of a person's needs, but there are boundaries that should be reserved for your lifelong mate to fulfill and not substitutes. I've found that it is nearly impossible to give what you never received and is why the Preparation phase (0–18?) of your life is very important to your emotional growth and development. No one had a perfect family, but some hindered the ability to get the essential elements that allowed a person to achieve emotional stability during the Separation (18–28?) and Independence (28–??) phases of life.

Why Do You Need Love, Acceptance, Appreciation, Respect, and Trust?

The five "Relationship Needs" for emotional survival:

1. Love (admiration)
2. Acceptance (understanding)
3. Appreciation (recognition)
4. Respect (honor)
5. Trust (honesty)

These needs can allow you to have more focus during your Separation and Independence phases of life. Without ample deposits into your five Relationship Needs accounts from your parents or other household members during the Preparation phase it is next to impossible to obtain the focus required to rise above mediocrity and truly take advantage of the opportunities that lie before you. If you look at each of these needs as joint-savings accounts that exist in all of your relationships, then you may be able to visualize how you may be able to improve the quality of your relationships (remember, it takes two to tango).

Relationship Needs Accounts

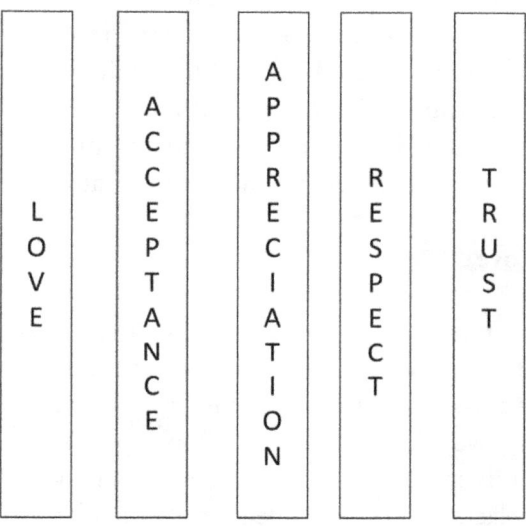

Figure 1-3

Your positive interactions (deeds and words) expressed in your relationships allow you to gain emotional assets. Over time, you build emotional assets by maintaining positive balances in your joint relationship needs accounts with others. When you have an emotional need, it will require the other person in the relationship to make a withdrawal from their emotional assets and make a deposit into the joint relationship needs account. Their giving should motivate you to make deposits in the joint relationship needs accounts. The challenge is having sufficient balances in your accounts so neither person feels they are doing all the work in the relationship (ever felt drained before?). Remembering that these accounts exists in all of your relationships with friends, family members, employer/supervisor, coworkers, subordinates, etc., can help you to understand your role in maintaining acceptable balances in your relationship needs accounts.

Children establish their initial relationship needs accounts during the Preparation phase of life with their parents or guardians. These initial relationship needs accounts will set the precedence for future relationships. A sign of their maturity is when children start giving back to those who made the initial deposits. The status of your relationship needs accounts at the end of the Preparation phase, will affect a person's ability to establish and maintain future healthy relationship needs accounts. Therefore, your relationship needs accounts can have a significant impact on your quality of life. I will discuss these Accounts in detail in the following paragraphs.

Number 1: Love

What is "love"? Love is the emotion that allows you to feel important, safe, and wanted. **Love is not sex**. Love can be expressed without any sexual interaction like it is in a normal child to parent, coworker, employer, friends, etc., relationships. Without love from immediate family members, a child is forced to look for love/admiration in other places such as extended family members, friends, gangs, team sports, youth groups, etc. There is a big difference between a person's decision to affiliate with a gang or a sports team. For most, the decision comes down to following the path of least resistance. I have discovered that people, like electrons, follow the path of least resistance when it comes to where people will go to find love, however pure or distorted. Unfortunately, most of the groups or people who offer the least amount of resistance are usually the most destructive and can negatively sway a person's value system or even physical safety!

Is Your Love Account Overdrawn?

Each one of us came into this world with empty relationship needs accounts and that includes the "love account." The responsibility to make the initial deposits in a child's "love account" lies with their parents. If they or acceptable stand-ins (grandparents, aunt, uncle, brother, sister, coach, teacher, etc.) do not make deposits in the child's "love account" through their selfless acts of love/admiration, a person can spend the rest of their lives trying to establish/maintain their "love accounts" in their relationships with coworkers, family, friends and spouse. Without at least one relationship that has a semiactive "love account," people expect someone else to do the impossible and that is to complete or fill them. If you ever wondered why an estimated 50% of marriages fail, you can look to the relationship's nearly empty "love and trust accounts" coupled with unmet or unrealistic expectations. There is a huge responsibility levied upon adults who desire to be parents, and that is to first develop and maintain love and trust accounts with their spouse prior to having children! Unfortunately for many, the children come before a stable relationship and that can determine whether or not the child starts out with at least a partially full-joint child and parent "love account." The status of the child and parent "love account" can mean for some the ability to focus on their goals or a life of misery. When the "love account" is almost empty, the quest for love consumes too many of their emotional and physical resources and may appear in the form of compulsive behavior.

Another aspect about love is that it is a verb and therefore, requires actions to make a deposit into another person's "love account." Saying "I love you" is not enough! Actions do speak louder than words. Acts of kindness without conditions, patience displayed with intent of listening, and time commitments (remember, time is nonrefundable!), and recognition of a person's value has the ability to make deposits to the "love account." Parents' unselfish expression of love to their children equips them to learn to love themselves because their love is reflected back to the child like the sun's rays striking the surface of the earth. Unfortunately for some their parent's reflection of love was obstructed by dark clouds of cruelty or selfishness and resulted in cold relationships.

A relationship between two people with almost empty "love accounts" will usually result in a "why can't you love me" tug of war that no one can win because neither person has a reserve capacity of love to give to their needy partner.

The ability to love yourself is an indicator of properly balanced "love accounts" and a person's ability to have fulfilling relationships. A fulfilling marital relationship is when two wholes come together verses two incompletes trying to do the impossible and that is making one from mismatched pieces. It is like trying to pour new wine into old wineskins, the two are not compatible and the end result is destructive for both the new wine and old wineskins. If a person's "love account" with parent(s) or guardian during the Preparation phase is empty because of neglect, it could spell trouble for their ability to have fulfilling relationships. Therefore, knowing and understanding your history and your potential mate's is important in determining if there will be future problems in the relationship. Bottom line is to get healthy before you start competing in the emotional Olympics.

Number 2: Acceptance

Did you ever do something that you thought was so horrible, when you were a child that you entertained the idea of running away only to find out that your absence would have caused more pain than your deed? Children need to know that they are accepted and wanted by their parents unconditionally. That does not mean that parents should not discipline their children, but it does means they should let their children know they are accepted and wanted unconditionally. Even if the pregnancy was unplanned, the child should not grow up hearing and thinking their entire life was a mistake! I believe conduct permitted is conduct taught, so the emphasis is on unconditional acceptance and not blanket approval of unacceptable behavior. The feeling of acceptance in the child to parent "acceptance account" allows a person to develop their self-confidence and self-esteem. When a person feels unconditionally accepted by their parent(s), they are comfortable with expressing their emotions and realize they are valuable and their birth was not a mistake. Caution—acceptance and approval are not interchangeable! I can accept that you are my child and a kleptomaniac but I don't have to approve of your behavior! Without acceptance, a relationship will never develop beyond physical passion and passion does not last. No one is willing to bare their soul to someone who does not accept or understand them. The key to developing intimacy hinges on the ability to feel accepted. Words of encouragement, positive reinforcement and acts of forgiveness after confession and reconciliation, can fill a person's "acceptance account."

I recommend each person acknowledge they have the potential to make valuable contributions to our society and they can choose to be an honorable and accepted member of humanity. As Dr. Seuss said, "To the world you may be one person; but to one person, you may be the world." Each person has the potential to have a place or a niche, but it requires personal discovery and an honest assessment of your strengths and weaknesses. Caution—if your attitude, which is reflected in your behavior, is truly deplorable, don't go walking around with rose-colored glasses! The people close to you may be rejecting you for valid reasons. You might be the one who needs to make a serious course correction, apologize and make restitution for past behavior. If you left home without that feeling of acceptance then it may be time to confess and seek reconciliation. If your parents do not restore your feelings of self-worth, after you have made earnest attempts to reconcile, then look for opportunities to be merciful toward others in your life and your labor of mercy will begin to fill your "acceptance/understanding" account with others.

Case in point, a close friend's son had a tough time finding acceptance from his mother. The issue he neglected to realize was that he had a tendency to publicly disrespect her and wounded her spirit. Unfortunately, he was acting out what he saw his father do to his mother. It was not until he saw the error of his ways and truly reconciled himself with her that he found the acceptance from her that he was longing for. Mind you, this did not happen overnight and it took years of work on his and her part. In the words of Saint Francis, "It is better to understand than to be understood." People are willing to accept you when you are willing accept responsibility for your actions.

Number 3: Appreciation

Some had parents who could not be pleased. Nothing was ever good enough. Being appreciated/recognized is important to gaining the ability to learn how to be needy. If you never felt appreciated you may find yourself trying to satisfy the needs of others, but yet feel guilty about expressing your needs. There is nothing wrong with being needy. Being thankful and expressing gratitude is one way to learn how to be content in your relationships because it prompts others to reciprocate by showing you their appreciation for your actions. If your partner does not respond to your expression of gratitude they are either selfish or you are operating with an overdrawn "appreciation account!" To remedy an overdrawn account, you are going to have to make a lot of deposits without the expectation of immediate withdrawals! In the case of the selfish person, your actions are going to have little to no influence on their behavior. To find the balance between giving thanks and receiving it in return, I recommend that you make a lot of deposits in the "appreciation account" so you will be entitled to make withdrawals during your time of legitimate need. If you have heard that you are selfish and only think of yourself from those who are close to you, then you are overdue on your evaluation of your ability to make others feel appreciated. Appreciation is also gained through recognition. For some people, the lack of appreciation/recognition is the primary reason why they chose to leave their current situation in hopes to find a place where they are appreciated. Finding appreciation is important and has the ability to inspire or reinforce good behavior.

Number 4: Respect

Ever wonder why respect is such a common demand from young people? Respect must be earned and it must be taught during the Preparation phase of life. In the past, one way young people learned respect was from their extended family. When children see their parents respecting their grandparents that allowed them to learn how to honor their elders and other authority figures. Some people became parents at a young age and instead of having parents who were equipped to provide the initial deposits into their "Respect Account" they were left with peers who were incapable of making deposits. Peer to peer like relationships between parent and child, usually result in relationships that do not have a high degree of respect. <u>Caution—*fear* and respect are not the same thing</u>! An environment where people are afraid is not healthy. Respect is expressing your views with reverence and acknowledgement of the value of the other person. If a child does not learn to respect and honor from their parents, then how is he/she to treat others who are in positions of authority? Respect has to be reciprocated in all relationships, to include the parent to child relationship. Lack of respect shown to either party will inhibit problem solving options, because respect affects trust.

Respect also has to do with your ability to feel Honored and children should show their parents "respect" by their desire to obey them. The Ten Commandments also directs us to respect and honor our parents and states, "Honor thy father and thy mother: that thy days may be long upon the land which the Lord thy God giveth thee" (Exodus 20:12).

Respect is needed in marital relationships and complements expressions of love. When either party is not respected (constant nagging, public and private ridicule, demeaning words or actions, etc.) it damages the relationship and no one wants to be close to someone who does not respect them. When you feel your opinion is valued or you are on par with your spouse and peers, it could encourage you to open up and bring your ideals to the table. Aristotle said, "No one can be a good commander unless he learns how to obey." Obeying is a by-product of respect. Leaders deserve to be respected and if you want to be a leader you have to learn how to respect those in authority. Without respect you should not expect to sit in a place of high authority that is unless you want to be a tyrant!

Number 5: Trust

Trust is one of mankind's basic instincts and exists at various levels in all of your relationships. When you first meet a person, your body's internal trust meter is trying to detect whether or not it is safe to be around that person. Parents showed their children how to trust by extending to them their resources and providing for their child's physical safety needs. If you grew up in an environment where you were not physically safe or experienced repeated breaches of honesty, trust in your relationships can be a big issue for you. When you did not experience trust in your parent to child relationship during the Preparation phase of life it could affect whether or not you blindly trust too early in your relationships, or defer to the opposite and or reluctantly extend your trust to anyone. Caution: Parents are their child's first teacher and that means you have to be honest with your children. Don't tell your children when the phone rings that you are not home. Be honest in your money transactions too! Regardless of their age, don't borrow money your child received as a gift, and not repay it. If you need the money, explain to your child why you had to use the money and why you are not in the position to repay it. It would be wise to use the money for something important and not to get your nails done or to go the bar! You build trust by being a responsible steward of your child's money. Your actions speak louder than words and will help your children know they are in a healthy, safe, and in a trustworthy environment. Hopefully, through relationships with honest people, you will learn to adjust your trust accordingly.

Trust in your relationships requires honesty. If you can't feel comfortable around someone, then that is an indication of a low level of trust and affects the ability to connect. If trust is not gained, it will usually result in avoidance and withdrawal. Remember, "trust accounts" exists in all relationships regardless of how brief (remember the last time you bought a car or played a carnival game?) In the initial stages of a relationship, you may extend your trust, but continue to verify until you learn about the other person's character. Trust is one of the reasons why people maintain their childhood relationships. When you have a long history of trust it supports your desire to connect and stay connected regardless of the physical distance. Without trust you don't have a relationship. When trust leaves a relationship there is a desperate need for confession, forgiveness, and reconciliation. Rebuilding trust in a relationship takes a lot of time and is hard work. Even after that, there is no guarantee the relationship will be restored to its initial luster and you cannot force the violated person to participate. Once trust is violated it takes away a corner stone from the very foundation of the relationship. Key to success is to be honest in your relationships and learn to be trustworthy, because if you can't be trusted, it is unreasonable for you to expect someone to extend their trust to you. Money can buy many things but it can't buy respect, reputation, or trust.

Getting First Things First ("Old Cart Before the Horse" Cliché)

Now that I discussed some of the issues that contribute to who we are, it is time to discuss another tragedy that ails people and that is trying to run before you crawl or walk! People who did not address the issues related to their inadequate relationship needs accounts should not believe they could go out and make their fortunes and have that ideal life they always dreamed of. If you think you can neglect sorting out emotional issues, let me ask you to consider the high cost in time (which is nonrefundable and priceless!) and money to support an addiction to alcohol, drugs, or other destructive compulsive behavior? Developing an addiction as a means to cope with the imbalances associated with not getting emotionally healthy is costly. All you have to do is look at the lives of materially-successful people who committed suicide, died due to drug overdose or are suffering with compulsive behaviors because their success did not complete them.

I also know you can't win a race by constantly looking in the rearview mirror! But every successful racer knows you have to spend some time in the garage and on the practice track before you compete on race day! I am not saying to do nothing until these issues are addressed, but to instead focus on making progress on your own emotional development so you can maximize your ability to recognize your limitations and capitalize on your opportunities related to your strengths. The Separation phase of life can be a time of personal awareness and growth. Making a commitment to personal growth and development, will allow you to use time as an ally verses a foe. If you think a mind is a terrible thing to waste, just think about the high cost of taking two steps forward and one step back! If you left home properly prepared, in other words, well-balanced relationship needs accounts with your family, friends, schoolmates, etc., then I encourage you to do whatever it takes to show them your sincere gratitude. It's the quality of our relationships and not material wealth alone that makes life worth living. Success is more gratifying when you are surrounded by people who genuinely love and support you.

CLEVELAND O. EASON

Personal Survival and Wellness

In my introduction (if you did not read my introduction, go back and read it now), I stated some of the people I initially came in contact with in my workplace environment during my early Separation phase of life were post-Vietnam era sailors. I have a lot of respect for Vietnam era veterans (my father served two tours in Vietnam and is a combat wounded veteran) and I acknowledge the sacrifices they made for our country. Unfortunately, when I joined the US Navy in the early 80's, our country did not value their sacrifices. Fortunately, that began to change after the first Gulf war. As such, some of them had lifestyles that would clash with today's military service expectations. Unfortunately for me, some of the people I worked for or chose to associate with, were not making good life choices. I was subjected to a post-seventies, work hard, play hard environment. Fortunately for me and our country, a new era began to emerge in the 1980s and the US Navy embraced policies such as a drug-free workplace, zero tolerance for gender and racial discrimination, personal accountability, and team building that helped to foster healthier learning and work environments. Don't get me wrong—our places of worship, military, schools or workplaces are not perfect, and never will be, but that does not mean we should not strive to improve those environments. During the Separation and Independence phases, your educational and/or work environment are where you spend the majority of productive hours and is also where you have most of your direct contact with other people. I can't understate the importance of finding a group of people worthy of your association (remember the path of least resistance?) Jeanne Mayo said, "Show me your friends and I will show you your future."

Finding people who can have a good time without external stimulants is a must. A mixed-gender group is helpful to allow you to have gender diversity in your relationships. Since you may or may not have a good picker, in other words, the ability to avoid following the path of least resistance, which can lead to finding people who will set you back in your progress, it may be necessary for you to avoid listening to natural instincts (which is hard!).

Remember, garbage in and garbage out, and greatness in and greatness out! If you are trying to renew your mind, you do not want reinforcement from environments that you know won't work. Developing a hobby, an interest in a cause, or volunteering are ways to meet people you may not normally associate with. Your local place of worship or other volunteer agencies are just a few examples of places to meet people or find information about groups that can provide the support you may be looking for.

The Internet is one place to find a listing for groups, but don't use chat rooms or social networking sites to replace the need to physically interact with people. The ability to look someone in their eyes allows you to determine their true sincerity (remember the trust meter). Within groups, you have the opportunity to meet some people who may be able to assist you in meeting the right people. I also encourage you to consider having a mentor. Preferably, your mentor should be someone who is at least ten to fifteen years older than you, successful in an area you desire growth and development, and will commit to not having a physical relationship with you. A mentor can understand where you are and where you are going and can help you create supportive alliances. A mentor is a person who wants to help you improve and should challenge you to forsake your destructive habits. Some friends will tolerate your destructive habits for the sake of companionship so there could be a rub between your mentor and your so-called friends. Caution mentors are not infallible, but if they are honest and sincere, they can help you gain some clarity about your future aspirations and possibly provide you some insight on making some important decisions. Ultimately, you are responsible for <u>ALL</u> of your decisions and you cannot blame anyone for your choices regardless of their level of influence. Dale Carnegie (twentieth-century multimillionaire) once said, "The difference between you today and you five years from now are the books you read and the people you meet." My 21st century update to Dale Carnegie's quote would include the music and podcasts you put in your ears and websites you browse. Your eyes and ears are the windows to your soul and therefore, you need to restrict what influences your inner thoughts. Because I agree with David A. Stoop "you are what you think." Bottom line, choosing your associates and friends is serious business and essential to your ability to experience progress during life's journey.

If you have not picked up on it by now, I believe you should spend your time in the late "Preparation" and early Separation phases of life identifying with who you are as an individual. Unfortunately, many young people get caught up in emotionally-draining personal relationships, become young parents, or develop compulsive-destructive behavior that inhibit or significantly delays their ability to focus on self-improvement and acquiring the skills they need to become emotionally and financially independent. I encourage you to avoid the temptation to get involved in negative environments that distract you from obtaining the educational and/or vocational training necessary to pursue worthwhile occupations or business ventures.

To answer the question about why you should concentrate on personal development during the Separation phase, I will share with you my philosophy about luck. Some say life is a matter of good or bad luck and I want to challenge you to adopt a different perspective. Good and bad things <u>will</u> happen in your life! Relying on luck means you are not accepting responsibility for what happens to you and sets you up to be a victim of circumstances! Luck is when preparation meets opportunity. For example, let's say you are a talented musician who dedicated five to eight hours a day to practicing and actively searching for opportunities. Finally, you discover an opportunity to audition for a band and are selected to be a member of the band that is going on a world tour (that happened to one of the individuals in my hometown!) What do you think the results would have been if you had a talent, but you never spent anytime practicing and actively searching for opportunities? Preparation allows you to take advantage of opportunities. If you never prepare, then you should not expect success to just drop in your lap! Therefore, luck is when preparation meets opportunity. If you don't use your time wisely to prepare for your future, which includes creating a vision of where you want to be, you will have to suffer the consequences of taking two steps forward and one step back, or even worse, one step forward and two steps back!

Chapter 2

Relationships
How Do You Manage Them?

We have all heard that behind every good man is an equally good woman and vice versa. What does this have to do with your personal road map to success or quality of life? Can your relationship with the right or wrong person equal the difference between poverty and wealth? I think so, but if you doubt me, history provides all the evidence I need to prove this theory. Ever heard of Raymond and Marie Fraietta Floyd, Gloria and Emilio Estefan or Bonnie and Clyde? Marie Fraietta Floyd's honest assessments of her husband, PGA golfer Raymond Floyd's performance, strengthened his mental toughness and contributed to his golf tournament wins. The story of Ronald and Nancy Reagan is a tale of a man who rekindled his fire due to his love affair with Nancy. History is riddled with stories of disastrous and successful couples that had their 15 minutes on the world's stage.

Initial Attraction

When I talked about love in the first chapter, I was preparing you to think about what determines your "right match." If you don't know your limitations or what's in your emotional seabag, then it will be hard for you to avoid finding love in "all the wrong faces and situations." Nothing is as gratifying as a relationship that is balanced, in other words, "equally yoked." My definition of "equally yoked" is the ability to be equally equipped to make deposits into each other's relationship needs accounts and the ability of the other person's strengths to complement/compensate for the other person's weaknesses. This creates two people capable of pulling the load with equal distribution of effort. On the contrast, nothing is more emotionally- and physically-draining than a relationship out of balance. No one person should have to do all the work when two people are available!

A close friend of mine was in a high-maintenance relationship (one in which the joint five relationship needs accounts were overdrawn) that took a severe toll on him emotionally and physically and resulted in him being forty pounds overweight. That might not sound like a lot of weight, but when you are not very tall, forty pounds can make a big difference! When he conceded to his wife's desire to end the relationship because of her commitment to a relationship with another man and "let go," he lost the forty pounds in just nine months and a couple of years later, met someone who was equally equipped to make deposits in their joint relationship needs accounts. Today, he is happier, healthier, and has a more balanced life. If you think marriage is not important to your future, then skip this chapter now and read it after your first divorce!

Does Age Really Matter?

I believe the quest for the right partner should not start if you are too young. What is considered to be too young? I believe that most people do not identify with who they are as a person until they are twenty-three to twenty-six years old and that applies to people who came from emotionally healthy families! Of course, there are exceptions to every rule, for example, if you have a childhood friend who has known you and you both have extensive knowledge of each other's personal background, marriage at an early age <u>might</u> result in a very compatible relationship. Even given those factors, you should know that there are big risks if both of you are not in the late Separation phase of life. Learning how to support yourself financially, without excessive involvement from your parents, occurs during the

Separation phase and is an important step in developing maturity and establishing realistic expectations. Even if you have not passed the Separation phase yet, read on, because developing a "clear mental vision" of the person you would like to partner with for the rest of your life cannot be understated; remember, there are exceptions!

Not to trivialize the incredible worth of a stable lifelong relationship, but I believe this analogy may be helpful. No one goes searching for a home without first defining what kind of home they want—a two-story colonial, one-story rancher, single-detached family, duplex, town house, neighborhood, budget, distance from work, etc. If you don't know what you want or what is important to you, then it's quite possible for the wrong person to get your attention. Relationships are not in the "go with the flow" category; in fact, the best things that life has to offer do not follow that philosophy. Knowing what you want is a sign of maturity and can help you avoid making a choice you will regret for the rest of your life (divorce does not erase the memories, emotional, and/or financial losses!) Some people do not know how to answer the "What do I want in a relationship?" question. How it is answered can have some long-term consequences.

Personal Radar: Is Yours Calibrated?

Why do we love who we love? Have you ever sat down and thought about what attracts one person to another? In my self-help stage of life (which I discovered is a never-ending process!) I discover that some people are either equipped or not equipped to make safe relationship choices. During World War II, the US Navy employed a new technology called Radio Detecting and Ranging, or radar. Radar was used to detect and provide the range of contacts. The radar operator still needed to use other information to determine if the contact was or was not a threat. During World War II and in the conflicts and wars that followed, the consequences of misidentifying a contact that was a threat as a non-threat, vice versa, had deadly consequences! I believe people have "personal radar" that detects potential romantic partners and like the radar the US Navy used during World War

II, it still needs an informed person to use their personal judgment to determine if they detected a good or bad match. From the pages of someone else's personal history, I will provide an example that describes the concept of "personal radar."

A close friend of mine after his first marriage (some refer to this as their "practice marriage") went through a phase when almost every woman he met was either married or very needy. It was like there was bait around his neck that only attracted women who were in tough situations. After his third relationship with a very needy woman (yes, it took him a while to wake up!), he realized it was not just the women who had issues, but he had issues he needed to work out. He discovered he needed to feel appreciated and as such, his "personal radar" was good at detecting needy people. People in disharmonious relationships can be rather needy. They were "I need a hero" relationships. His need to feel appreciated coupled with his fear of long-term relationships due to the failure of his first marriage led to bad choices.

The dangers of adulterous relationships are too numerous to state, and since we are all basically farmers who reap what we sow, I don't want to encourage anyone to have a relationship with another person's spouse. The law of the harvest has terrible repercussions for those who don't obey and respect it! So why the story? It was used to illustrate a point and that is you need to know what you want, before you go searching and more importantly, you need to know your vulnerabilities. If you want success in life, it starts with knowing yourself.

Do You Know Your Radar Limitations?

If you wonder why you're involved with who are with now, take a look at your childhood and the role models who guided you. Who showed you what it is like to have a loving and supportive relationship? Children who lived through their parent's disastrous marital or live-in arrangements often struggle as adults to obtain healthy relationships. Sometimes, if we have deficiencies, a well-balanced person can lead us to the road to health. I wouldn't want you to put that burden on anyone because I believe you should resolve personal issues prior to the relationship instead of in the relationship. Remember the "personal radar" story!

The swimmer analogy applies to whether or not you may be healthy enough to let someone help you overcome some unresolved issues. I will begin with a question. If you are a weak swimmer and someone needs help what do you do? Do you swim out and risk both of you drowning or do you call for help and provide assistance from ashore? If you answered, called for help and provided assistance from ashore, then maybe an independent, sensitive and emotionally stable person could possibly help guide you to the road to independence (remember Ronald and Nancy Reagan?) Acknowledging your weaknesses is critical, but there are a lot of people who are caught up in the fog that prevents them from seeing they have a problem (the ol' can't see the forest for the trees problem.)

If you're a person who lacks clarity of your own issues, you would have swum out and tried to be a hero and found yourself ill equipped to carry out the task. In the swimmer analogy as with personal relationships the results could be tragic for the all involved!

You should question your initial attractions especially if you have a history of involving yourself in bad relationships. People who know you and truly care for you; and are without selfish motives, can be great resources for helping you avoid collisions due to defective radar! Relationships do not fall in the category of "If at first you don't succeed try, try again," inventions do, but not people.

If at First You Don't Succeed…

One way friends try to comfort each other after a failed relationship is to say, "There are plenty of fish in the sea," which can lead you into the "try, try, try again" trap. Failed relationships require time for self-reflection which is why I'm always puzzled by the bumper sticker that say "My ex rides a broom". If that is true, then what does that say about you? If you can't figure it out, then I strongly recommend that you consult with a counselor who can assist you in your analysis. Bottom line is, you can't change someone else; you can only provide them your influence, which they can choose to reject. The only person you can change is you and changing yourself is hard work, especially if you don't have a moral conscience as a reference point in your decision-making! If you don't change or calibrate your "personal radar" then the people you allow to be part of your inner circle won't change either.

After reading the proceeding paragraphs, you have probably concluded that I don't have much confidence in love at first sight. Initial attraction is typically a poor indicator and may result in many years of disappointment and heartbreaks. Having a clear vision of what you want in a relationship is important to identifying the characteristics your future mate should possess. If the initial attraction allows you to go deeper and discover the qualities that you were looking for, then congratulations, but if further examination reveals characteristics you are not willing to live with for the rest of your life, then it's time to say goodbye before you consummate your commitment in a sexual or marital relationship.

Happily Ever After?

Going back to the five relationship needs that everyone needs to feel loved, accepted, appreciated, respected, and trusted is why they are needed to establish and maintain relationships. Regardless of how independent you are, you need relationships with family, friends, and if married, your spouse. No one person can satisfy all of your needs, which is why having a healthy balance between family, friends, and spouse can help ensure you are capable of sustaining those relationships in their respective priorities and importance. If you are wondering what priority you should place on your relationships, your first priority should be to your marital relationship. If the other relationships do not respect the precedence of your marital relationship, then the sincerity of those relationships should be in question. Example, if you and your spouse work and only have time together on evenings and weekends, your family and friends should respect your need to reconnect after your time of separation. A family member or friend that stops by unannounced shortly after you arrive from work on a regular basis and stays for hours on end is not respecting your relationship and the need to reconnect with your spouse. The marital relationship is the nucleus, the center of all your other relationships and therefore, the choice of your marital partner is one that should not be taken lightly.

Finding the right person requires you to look beyond the initial physical attraction, looks are somewhat important, but just like your other long-term decisions, you must go beyond the surface and dig deeper. To allow the relationship to develop beyond passion requires intimacy. No one should sign a thirty-year mortgage and neglect to have a home inspection that could uncover some major problems! The details of the relationship that go beyond initial physical attraction are essential to the development of companionate love which requires intimacy. You can't have intimacy without balanced "relationship needs" accounts. The problem a lot of couples have is they begin a sexual relationship without considering the state of their joint relationship needs accounts.

Relationships 101

Before you can be a couple, you have to first go beyond the initial attraction. I am going to use an analogy to describe the relationship development process. Imagine, if you will, that each of your relationships, whether with acquaintances or your future spouse is a house with four rooms. There are a couple of rules that apply to this house. Rule number one, is before you can advance to next room, it requires both people to open their door. Consider it like a room with two sliding doors that equally cover the entrance to the next room. You can slide your door open, but if the other person refuses to open their door, then you don't advance to next room. Rule number two, the other person can leave the room and go back to the previous room or leave the house altogether without your consent! This rule gives credence to why the spouse is sometimes the last to know the other person has decided to leave the relationship! Now that you know the rules, let's take a look at the relationship house.

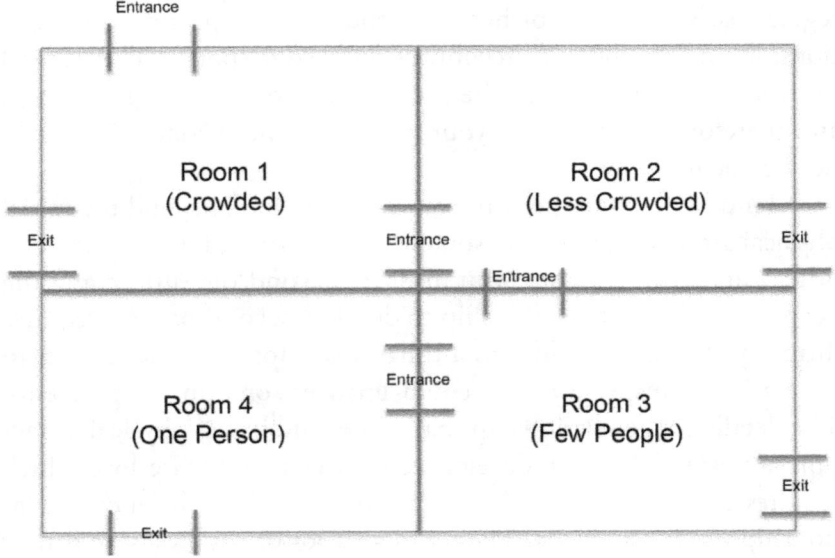

Figure 2 - 1

Room 1

Room 1 should be the safest room in the house! It is where you first meet. This is where basic information exchange occurs, your name, profession, etc., and where you eventually develop the ability to distinguish each other in a crowd. Think of this like a place you would meet someone to sell your Craigslist item. It's public, it's safe, and if there is trouble, you easily get help. Another aspect of this house, which is true for all rooms in this house, is that it has an emotional and physical layer in each room. Remembering rule 2, you can leave without the other person's permission. Therefore, each person has the freedom in room 1 to walk out without revealing very much of themselves. As it should be, room 1 is reserved for sharing of information that will result in little to no risks. In the later stages of room 1, where after meeting a couple of times by chance and both have decided it's time to move to room 2, and to facilitate this, you exchange telephone numbers. Caution: If the person you are with in room 1 starts making assertive demands for your undivided attention, you may be involved with someone who is very needy. If they are in a rush to occupy a majority of your time, they probably have some unresolved deficiencies. Time spent in room 1 could be indefinite and depends on the level of mutual interest. A suggested time frame could be two to three weeks. Taking it slow can give you a green or a red light on whether or not you are willing to take the risks associated with going to room 2.

Room 2

Remembering rule 1, that no one advances to the next room unless both parties open their door is when you discover that entering room 2 means opening yourself up to some limited but manageable risks. In room 2, because you have exchanged contact information, you can agree to meet over coffee or a Dutch meal (both parties pay for their own meals; sorry, guys, even when a girl says she's okay with paying for her own meal, deep down inside, she probably expects and wants you to pay the tab) with neither one of you losing much if the relationship does not to go any further.

In order to avoid unrealistic expectations, you need to be reasonable in your expenditures during the early stages of a relationship. Money can't buy you love and if you are exhausting all of your financial resources on a new acquaintance, it will affect your financial stability and possibly build resentment in the relationship. Don't be too cheap! Despite the demands for equality, most women expect you to pay when you invite them out for a date! If you don't pay, even if they agreed in advanced to "going dutch," she may conclude that you are stingy and not the one they want to pursue in a relationship. To minimize letdowns, it would be beneficial to make sure your dates are within your financial limits. In room 2, you don't mind the other person knowing more personal information about you and they don't mind sharing their personal information. Personal information should still be limited but emotions should be authentic and genuine. The relationships you have with coworkers, classmates, i.e. people you have frequent or daily contact with, will normally reside in room 2. You know each other, but you still limit information that you divulge because you do not expect to develop deep or lifelong relationships with that person or have reasonable expectation of confidentiality. Activities in room 2 should include time with your friends to find out whether or not your new interest can tolerate them.

Time spent in room 2 depends on you and the other person's interest in you. It could be a couple of weeks, months or indefinitely. Room 2 is also where you find out about the level of enthusiasm the other person has for you. If they are too busy or have little time to get together for a short date, then it is safe to say the relationship won't advance farther than room 2. The best way a person can show their interest in you is by setting time aside for you. You have to be reasonable and inquire when is the best time to contact them, but believe me if they are interested, it should be relatively obvious. The level of mutual interest you and your acquaintance have in each other will determine if and when you will transition to room 3. The decision to move to room 3 is where the real risks occur.

Room 3

Room 3 is where you are comfortable with letting the other person know where you live and would allow them to visit you at your residence. Phone calls, texts, etc., and interest in day-to-day activities in the early phases of the relationship occur frequently and are freely initiated by both people involved in the relationship. You share information about yourself when you know the other person will honor your need for privacy and or confidentiality. Lifelong friends and your fiancé are examples of people who will occupy space in room 3. Understanding the extent of comparable relationships that occupy this room should allow you understand the level of closeness, confidentiality, shared experiences and trust that should exists if your dating relationship is truly in room 3. Your conversations should not just be text messages and should consist of real, in person (preferred) or via telephone, audible conversations if you are in room 3. Caution, if you think you are in room 3, you may be in the room by yourself if the other person does not reciprocate the same level of interest or responses!

Room 4

Once you have entered room 4, you need to assure you really know who the other person is and whether or not they are in the same room as you on the emotional level! Room 4 should be reserved for your spouse and no one else because this is where you are the most vulnerable. There are very few secrets, besides the ones that are reserved for the degree of privacy to allow that level of mystique that should exist in every marital relationship (e.g. how does she do that trick with her hair?) Since room 4 is reserved for your spouse, it is also where sexual activities occur. You are the most vulnerable in room 4, and as such you should understand the consequences that go along with being vulnerable. It is in room 4 that you share your dreams for aspirations, secret fears, physical, and sexual needs. If you progressed through the relationship house with maturity and mental clarity, then you won't regret allowing the relationship to progress to room 4, if you rushed, someone you really don't know might be in your most private space! It's like letting the enemy walk into your very bedroom.

Obstacles to Good Judgment

If you keep the "relationship house" analogy in mind, you can see why abstaining from sex or delaying it in your relationship is strongly recommended. For some, a first date, dinner, and sex relationship may sound exciting, but the ability to provide long-term satisfaction is quite doubtful. The first date, dinner, and sex relationship is when people go from room 1 to room 4 at the physical level without thinking about the risks they are taking. Trust is often very low in room 1 to room 4 relationships because of "if you had sex with me on the first date, what is to stop you from having sex with someone else on the first date" mentality. Jealousy is an emotion that often runs rampant in room 1 to room 4 relationships. If you have ever experienced jealousy as a recipient or deliverer, then you have a basic understanding of why trust is important in your relationships!

Jealous people usually have low self-esteem and/or have experienced relationships where trust was violated. The fear of being betrayed and the feeling of loss may cause bad behavior like interrogations and implied ownership rights. No one owns you and you don't own anyone because healthy relationships exist because there is a mutual desire to maintain a connection and not because of fear, intimidation or servitude (noticed that each room had an exit). This does not mean you do not have the right to expect the other person to exhibit conduct that is conducive to the relationship and demonstrate their commitment.

A person's sense of obligation should be because of their character and not because of fear caused by physical intimidation and/or economic dependency related to Neanderthal behavior. Being in love, means that both people value the relationship and that there will be a sense of loss if the five relationship needs accounts are being overdrawn. Expressing concerns about potential loss due to inappropriate behavior is not jealously and is expected because silence means approval. If one person is trying to be the gatekeeper and makes statements such as "who is that," "why do they call," etc., it may be because there is a lack of trust in their mate's sense of judgment when it comes to choosing friends, or it could be a sign of jealously and/or a desire to control or dominate, and none of the above are acceptable!

The risks people take in room 1 to room 4 relationships are not just emotionally but can be physical as well. The dangers of sexually transmitted diseases, emotional and physical trauma, or an unplanned pregnancy can be devastating. It should not come as a surprise that passion fades quickly in these types of relationships because they never took the time to graduate to the next room on the emotional level. Unfortunately, some people make their marital choices based on the room 1 to room 4 scenarios. And when the passion fades, consider looking for the lost passion in the arms of another lover, making the same mistake all over again. If the relationship never matured because sex was confused with love, then you can expect trouble in the future. Bottom line, make sure you understand the risks you take by moving too fast because the consequences can threaten life itself.

Family and Friends

What about family and friends? How can they help you develop your relationships? Going back to "personal radar," those who are close to you that do not have selfish motives can possibly identify some compatibility issues neither one of you ever thought about. Some words of caution about selfish motives and that is, not all the people you categorize as friends live up to the obligations associated with true friendship. Your friends may have fears about loss of intimacy (remember, close friends occupy space in room 3) and time once reserved to them and may not be forthcoming or honest with their advice. Exposing your relationship to family and friends may allow them to see if your potential mate is in the same room that you are in. Your vision could be blurred because you are too close to the situation (inability to see the forest for the trees).

When your vision is not clear, it is possible for others to help you adjust your vision through their observations. Family approval does not guarantee you will have a happy relationship, but if your family and friends have concerns, it would be in your best interest to validate whether or not their concerns are warranted.

Bad Tree, Bad Fruit?

Sorting out your past is very important and usually does not come to fulfillment until after or during the late Separation phase of life. Your emotional and financial stability can significantly affect the quality of your relationships, and therefore, I recommend delaying the decision to marry until you have successfully transition through or are in the late the Separation phase of life. As stated previously, in Separation phase you learn how to support yourself without excessive involvement from your parents and unless you have both sorted out your issues or at least identified them, it is unreasonable to expect to have a fulfilling relationship in room 3 or room 4.

As stated previously, in Chapter 1, a relationship between two people with almost empty "love accounts" will normally result in tug-of-war because each person is trying to get what the other does not have to share. You can't get blood from a turnip and you can't pour from an empty cup! A good indicator to consider before opening your side of the room 4 door is, "What kind of relationship did he/she have with their parent(s)?" A woman who has a loving and supportive relationship with her father is usually capable of expressing herself with confidence and has a high degree of self-esteem. Typically, she is comfortable with extending her trust to a compatible man. Her value and self-worth were established and reinforced during her childhood and she does not need to sacrifice her values to find acceptance; in other words, play at sex for love. Likewise, a man who had a loving and supportive relationship with his mother generally has a high degree of respect for women and is usually comfortable with expressing and sharing his emotions.

When you are considering a relationship with a lifelong partner, your family trees may have significant influence on the ability to have mutually satisfying relationships (you can't breed a dog with a tiger!) and the health of your future children. There are exceptions, but it is unwise to completely ignore past history. A good tree typically bears good fruit. For a person to overcome their past they need to either have: strong personal character traits, experienced the intervention of positive role models, had a spiritual awakening, or any combination of the above. In situations where the person broke the "bad tree, bad fruit" mold, family approval and acceptance is usually unobtainable and probably should not be pursued.

The mate selection process is critical and I believe the reason why many marriages fail is because of poor mate selection criteria and not acknowledging that relationships take time to develop. "Happily ever after" doesn't mean there won't be challenges, but it begins with you and whether or not you and your future spouse are prepared to accept the responsibilities of a lifelong commitment. A mature person has the ability to recognize their strengths and weaknesses and they have the courage to walk away if they cannot accept the other person "as is" before the marriage. The decision to walk away should be before the commitment to marry and not six months after you said your vows! One of my shipmate's marriage lasted only 48 hours when the bride refused to go on the honeymoon! Once you are married, you must commit to respectfully resolve your issues. A harmonious lifelong relationship is the best environment for raising children. Raising children in a combative environment, will most likely result in bad tree bearing bad fruit scenario.

Common Relationship Pitfalls

So what do you do if you are already sexually active in your premarital relationship? Be extremely careful, especially if you spent short periods of time in rooms 1, 2, and 3! Your sense of judgment might be severely flawed and allow you to introduce errors. The illusion of good sex for some is the driving factor in maintaining their relationships. Unfortunately, this is true for both genders. I recommend to look beyond sex and to ask yourself, "How does this person fulfill my five relationship needs?", "Is this person equipped to make deposits in our joint relationship needs accounts?", "what is our ability to communicate and resolve differences?", and "would I want this person to raise my children?" If sex is all you share, then you are in trouble because sex is not love. If all you have in common before the relationship is legalized is time in the sack, do you think a piece of paper is going to provide fidelity and trust? Every successful relationship requires the ability to express desires, dreams and feelings. Arriving at the conclusion that you have a shallow relationship is difficult for some people who enjoy the sex, but don't want to risk losing their relationship because the other issues are just too hard to talk about. If you are involved in a relationship like the one I just described, then I encourage you to reevaluate your mate-selection criteria.

It's Your Decision

When two people publicly state their marital intentions too soon, then the planning for the big day can foreshadow some of the basics like, "Should we really get married!" If you want a relationship that is going to last you need to experience authenticity and the ability to work through differences. That doesn't happen overnight, it takes time to develop an authentic relationship. A priest I know said he preferred performing funerals over weddings. The reason why he preferred funerals was because, unlike marriages, at least everyone knew what to expect when the ceremony was over! (John is dead, and he is not coming home after the funeral!) Marriage is hard work and requires a long-term commitment and resolve to thrive vice just to survive! If you think marriage will subdue jealousy (usually caused by lack of trust and/or low self-esteem) or quell compulsive behavior (alcoholism, dishonesty, drug use, gambling, etc.), you're wrong! In most cases, marriage results in those negative attributes, such as jealously or compulsive behavior to intensify into a "Welcome to My Nightmare" situation. This is especially true when the other person does not accept responsibility for their behavior and gets help (remember the swimming rescue story!) Success in marriage requires two emotionally healthy people committed to a lifelong relationship.

Have Invitations Will Marry?

Don't get caught up in the hype that a good wedding makes a good marriage. I have seen too many people have a beautifully-planned wedding that produced a nightmare of a marriage (remember the priest who preferred funerals!) Give your relationship some time to grow by slowing progressing through the "relationship house." Taking it slow, will allow you to determine whether or not your five relationship needs accounts (love, acceptance, appreciation, respect, and trust) can be maintained in your relationship. When both people feel that their five relationship needs accounts are being properly maintained, then you have a foundation to build upon. The decision to marry requires two people to commit and live up to the decision. Therefore, the decision to marry is one-half yours and one-half your fiancé, but not your caterer, dressmaker, family, or friends. You will both be responsible for your decision, if there are cold feet, it is necessary to address those concerns during premarital counseling.

There may be some valid reasons for your cold feet or some issues that you need help understanding before the marriage. Even if you don't have cold feet, I strongly recommend premarital counseling before you announce or set your wedding date. Premarital counseling will allow you both to discuss some of those issues related to marriage without the pressure of a wedding date and could allow to you both to address some issues you may have overlooked.

Case in point, a close friend of mine married his college sweetheart and five years into the marriage, he discovered his wife never had any intentions on having children. Although she expressed her feelings about having children before they married, he thought he could change her mind after they were married. Unfortunately, he was wrong and that issue eventually resulted in the end of their marriage. It might sound like I am stating the obvious but you would be surprised about the issues couples overlook before making their final wedding plans.

Conflict Management

Another common misconception is that if there are no disagreements before the marriage then life together will be harmonious. The same priest who said he preferred funerals over weddings also said, "You should not marry anyone unless you have had at least one big disagreement." His reasoning is that you need to know what is your and your future spouse's capacity to forgive and you need to develop problem-solving skills. I'm not saying to be argumentative, but I am saying you should feel free to express your feelings, even if you know the other person may disagree. If you feel like you are walking on eggshells, in other words the other person is very sensitive about various discussion topics, before you are married, just image the tragedy after the marriage. Additionally, if you have not had at least one disagreement, then it is quite possible one of you is masquerading and avoiding being authentic about their feelings. The dating process for some is when they exercise their best behavior and do not reveal their true personality until after the marriage (welcome to my nightmare syndrome). That is why I recommend premarital counseling and why it is important to be authentic so you can determine whether or not you and your future spouse have the tools to overcome your differences and build on your commonalities. Remember, your spouse is your personal confidant who will reside in room 4 and is entitled to know the real you. Because conflict management is essential in your ability to maintain positive relationships with your spouse, family, friends, and co-workers, I have included some conflict management tips. (Hint: In order to apply these tips to your other relationships, just replace spouse with co-worker, family or friend.)

Conflict Management Tips

1. Don't use physical intimidation. One of you has the physical advantage and the use of physical intimidation does not help to reduce tension or encourage cooperation and will result in loss of respect and trust.
2. Focus on the issue, not the other person. For illustration purposes, let's suppose a married couple has one car and their spouse is (three days out of five) twenty minutes late picking him or her up from work. One approach to addressing this issue would be the following dialogue:
"I know we agreed that you would pick me up from work at 4:30. Since there is difficulty meeting that schedule, I recommend that you pick me up at 5:00, what do you think?"
Ending with a question and using "I" verses "you" allows the other person to hear your concerns about the *issue*, hear your *recommendation* and finally let them know you are open to their *suggestions*. If they would have said, "You are always late picking me up! Can't you be on time?" Instead of encouraging their spouse to help develop an acceptable compromise, the spouse was put on the defensive and it can quickly become a test of wills, vice problem solving.
3. Don't talk down, instead talk peer to peer. No one likes to be talked down to. In order to maintain your relationships, you should avoid creating a master to slave conversation

style. Your spouse is a co-contributor to your relationship needs accounts and lifelong partner whose input deserves to be respected and valued.

4. Be willing to see things from the other person's perspective or view. When you forget to consider the issue from the other person's perspective, you could be blinding yourself to some very important information. Using the late pickup from work scenario as an example, maybe it was unrealistic for either one of them to think their spouse could pick them up each day at 4:30 because they get off work at 4:00 and distance of their job to their place of employment, plus traffic will inevitably result in unavoidable delays.

5. Listen attentively first and without interruptions—talk later. I can't understate the value of being a good listener! When someone is explaining an issue to you, give the other person your undivided attention (not a good time to check your smartphone to update your online status!) It is also helpful to learn to develop patience and paraphrase what you heard the other person say. When the other party knows you actually heard and understand their side of the story, it can be a breaking point in problem solving. Most conflicts can be resolved once both parties actual understand the issue.

6. Avoid "I'm right, you're wrong." When you develop a self-righteous attitude and refuse to listen because you think you are right and they are wrong, it is unrealistic to think it will be possible to reconcile your differences. Additionally, if they are wrong and accept their fault, no one that I know wants to be constantly reminded of their fault.

7. Think before you speak. The tongue is a double-edged sword! It is a lethal weapon that can inflict as much damage on you as it does the other person. This is contrary to what the nursery rhyme says (sticks and stones may break my bones but words will never hurt me—that's a big lie!) Remember words echo in a person's memory and if you think before you speak, you can save yourself from damaging or destroy-

ing a relationship with coworkers, family, friends or spouse. Spoken words like bullets cannot be recalled.
8. Think long-term vice now. If you don't consider the long-term consequences of not coming up with a viable solution to your issue, you could be in for a hard road ahead. Unresolved issues create resentment and without resolution can result in the loss of intimacy (you've lost that loving feeling) and bitterness.
9. Establish ground rules for expressing anger prior to discussing issues. Here are a few recommendations:
   a. Acceptable cool-off period. If tempers flare, allow each person the space they need to calm down so it will be easier to choose to respond vice react. High emotion results in low logic. Thirty to forty-five minutes is adequate, if both parties choose not to engage each other physically or verbally during that time of separation. Don't abuse this tool! I know of people who used arguments as a tool to get out of the house and party with friends.
   b. Agree to reconvene. Sometime issues come up at a time when it is not appropriate to discuss them. If you are on the verge of an extreme debate, it may be necessary to agree to discuss the issue at a later date and time and live up to that commitment without putting it off for another day. For example, my ex-wife chose to argue with me over an entry in the checkbook while I was driving in my uncle's funeral procession. Needless to say, I was not emotionally prepared to discuss the issue and it was appropriate to delay discussion of that issue.
   c. Agree not to shout or use profanity. Enough said.
   d. Agree not to bring up past arguments. Let past disagreements remain in the past. If you addressed the issue in the past, let the lesson learned exist, but let the resolved issue or mistake to remain in the past.
   e. Agree not to use of alcohol or drugs. Being mentally impaired because of alcohol or drug use is extremely

dangerous and should not be tolerated. When people resort to the use of alcohol or drugs during disagreements they may have an addiction and are using the argument as an excuse to exhibit their compulsive behavior.

f. Agree not to use physical violence. Related to 1, but I want to state you both need to agree not to use violence to express anger or frustration. Even if the one person is physically smaller than the other, that does not mean they cannot inflict bodily harm or destroy personal property. Physical violence is not acceptable and creating an environment of fear (destruction of personal property or inflicting injury) has never provided long-term solutions to differences due to loss of respect and trust. Remember respect and fear are not interchangeable. Violence reduces trust and raises concerns for personal safety.

10. Be the first to forgive and forget. Related to 9d except it added the element of forgiveness. If you have chosen to forgive by accepting the other person's apology, and if necessary restitution, you are also under the obligation to work toward setting the past aside. If you are the one who needs to say you are sorry, it is important to look the person in their eyes (if that is acceptable in your culture) so they can see your sincerity and intent to move beyond the past violation. Finally, don't wait for the other person to make the move before you begin to reconcile, instead you make the first move. Most people want to avoid conflict and when you demonstrate your ability to forgive by taking the first step, it will usually result in the other person's increased enthusiasm to communicate and collaborate with you.

11. Learn to confess and reconcile. Confessing that you made a mistake and actively choosing to refill the relationship needs accounts is important to the vitality of your relationships. Saying "I'm sorry" is not enough. I will use the table and nail analogy as visualization for the need for restitu-

tion. Picture if you will a beautiful mahogany table that has numerous big nails driven in it. The nails represent the injury, whether emotional or physical or both, that you did to someone else. Saying "I'm sorry" is equivalent to pulling the nails out of the wood, it leaves behind holes that have to be repaired. Restitution is act of filling in the holes and refinishing the wood after you caused injury.

I can't over express the importance of having good problem solving skills. Without them, your relationship's with, spouse, family, friends and co-workers, five relationship needs accounts will be severely overdrawn and have little to no chance of being restored.

Foreign or Domestic? The Issue of Language

Being a man who has had the privilege of traveling to foreign countries, I realize there are times when people consider having a long-term relationship with a foreigner (yes, Americans can be foreigners too!) While in France, I met an American woman who left her loving and supportive family in Arizona and at the time, lived happily with her husband of more than twenty years and their three children in France. There are countless examples of people who have forsaken their homeland in the name of love. In relationships between foreigners, some couples may have to overcome the "language" hurdle as well as all of the previously-stated issues pertaining to emotions, relationships, and conflict management. If you have ever taken dance lessons, then you can probably relate to following analogy.

Language, like dance, requires someone to accept the role as teacher and the other as follower. If you are a student, then you need to humbly follow the lead of the teacher in order to successful learn a new dance step. It does not mean that the student does not have anything to offer, but if student does not follow the teacher, then it will be impossible to develop oneness and be in step without stepping on a lot of toes! This lead follow principle applies to role of a foreign language in a relationship. If one of you does not have superior language skills in the other person's literate language, it will be frustrating to establish any meaningful conversations and develop a deep relationship.

Secondly, the person who has superior language skills, ideally should be extremely fluent in the dominant language of the country you decide to live in. For example, if you are an American who decides to establish a relationship with someone who lives in France and cannot read or speak French, it will be very difficult for you to have an effective relationship, if the other person does not have the ability to successfully translate from French to English and vice versa both orally and written. Conversations will be limited by ability of the speaker of the dominant country's language translation skills. Using the American dwelling in France example, if her husband's English is at the third-grade level, then it would be unrealistic to think conversations will exceed that level if one of them did not make a significant effort to bridge the gap. Fortunately for her, she was fluent in French and successfully transitioned over the language hurdle. Without appropriate language skills, all the other issues related to compatibility will be significantly strained.

Ideally, the individual who does not speak the country's dominant language should be assisted and encouraged to learn to read, speak, and write, in other words, become fully literate in the country's language. One of the biggest obstacles for adults who want to learn a new language is the fear of being humiliated when they try to communicate in the foreign language (yes, English for some is a foreign language!) The proficient speaker of the country's dominant language should create an environment where the individual is encouraged by correction and guidance without harshness. Speaking louder and with more intensity does nothing to improve the other person's ability to understand what you are saying (illiteracy does not cause hearing loss!) Development of a safe atmosphere greatly enhances their ability to gain language proficiency. The foreigner should be encouraged to take language classes as this will help in their assimilation into their new environment.

Patience on the part of the proficient speaker will allow the other person to communicate without interruptions instead of completing their mate's words when they encounter difficulty, especially in public settings, communicating an emotion or ideal in the foreign language. Allowing the other person to speak for themselves could reduce the likelihood of the proficient speaker becoming a "crutch" which can lessen their desire to develop language proficiency. Developing language proficiency will also alleviate extreme dependencies on the native speaker and allow the foreigner (which could be you!) to have independence and self-esteem in their new homeland. Nothing is more frustrating than having advanced educational skills and lacking the ability to express your emotions, needs and thoughts orally or in written form! Just imagine if you have children and only one of you has the necessary language skills to properly tutor your children or help with their homework assignments. No one wants to feel that they have little to contribute to the relationship and without appropriate language skills it can be very frustrating for all parties involved.

Assimilation Factors

There are a lot of issues people do not consider when deciding to relocate a foreigner to their country or choosing to immigrate abroad. One issue that can be difficult to overcome, is failing to consider the bond they may have with their family and friends. All things considered, if they left home with well-balanced relationship needs accounts (love, acceptance, appreciation, respect, and trust), they will need to stay connected with their family and friends. Personal history is just as important in the selection of a foreign born spouse, as it is for a domestic spouse. Information about their relationship with parents and siblings, whether or not he/she experienced the Separation phase, relationship history, education and language skills should be ascertained and will impact on the quality of the relationship.

At a glance, it might seem I am stating the obvious, but I have known many couples that failed to acknowledge these issues. I have known people (mostly men) who made their decision to marry a foreigner after meeting them on a holiday or port visit (room 1 to room 4 relationships.) The added strain of language (remember, without language proficiency, a person can feel belittled) coupled with feeling socially isolated due to being far away from family and friends, could make life far away from home very difficult. Some people marry a person who came from an economically-disadvantaged situation thinking that money can buy them love and we all should know the answer to that question is a firm no!

If you decide to marry a foreigner, a budget to return with them to their homeland, high-speed internet, and long distance telephone calls must become part of your normal expense budget. If your foreign spouse has a strong desire to frequently return home without you, it could be a signal that something else is going on, especially if marriage was primarily for economic reasons. Agreeing in advance to develop a reasonable allowance to support these expenses is a must and cannot be ignored. I also recommend that you seek out a community or organization comprised of people from their homeland so they can communicate with others in their native tongue, hence reducing the feeling of isolation. You will need to make adjustments and accept various aspects of their culture. It would be unreasonable for you to expect them to be the only to go through cultural adjustments.

The cost of immigration, potential to provide financial support to family members residing in their homeland, frequency of contact (visits, telephone, email, etc.), and desire to relocate to your country have to be discussed explicitly so you both have a complete understanding of the emotional and financial commitments. Initially, they may not be able to contribute financially to the household and may depend on you solely for financial support. In this situation, I recommend that you establish a joint account that provides them equal access to the household's budget so they don't feel like a child every time there is a financial need. I also strongly suggest there should be open dialogue to encourage active participation in planning and executing the household budget.

A foreign-born spouse may desire to reenter the work force. If you decide to live in America, you should know some employers requires proof of a high school degree or its equivalent, a general education degree (GED), before allowing the person to be eligible for training or positions of increased authority. Just imagine how difficult it would be for you to pass a high school equivalency exam using your secondary language! Identifying with this educational challenge can help you to appreciate the need for excellent multilingual skills and your responsibility to assist them to improve their language proficiency through enrollment in language classes, compassionate tutoring and social activities.

There are other issues about in the "foreign or domestic" decision, such as compatibility of values (family, finances, religion, etc.) that may exist and create conflict. Language proficiency combined with temperance and tolerance hold the keys to determining whether or not the couple will be able to overcome the barriers that prevent the development of oneness without a complete sacrifice of individuality. Not to discourage anyone from having a relationship with a foreigner, because you never know where your true love may come from, but it is unrealistic to think you can ignore language skills or issues related to assimilation and how they can challenge a couple's ability to develop intimacy and oneness. If you do not have patience and a genuine interest in the other person's culture and language, then you will not be able to establish the oneness needed to have both a compatible and successful relationship.

I have seen a lot of miserable unions between foreigners and their new country's natives and conversely, I have also seen wonderfully loving relationships between foreigners. Both parties must consider the assimilation and language factors before making a decision that could spell emotional and financial ruin due to ignorance!

Practice Marriage?

Unfortunately, a high number of first marriages end in divorce. In fact, some people consider them for training purposes only! Marriage requires a lifelong commitment between two emotionally-healthy mature adults prior to the marriage. The relationship requires room to discern whether or not it will be healthy enough to develop into a viable long-term relationship. A viable long-term relationship is when your love has evolved to the stage where you enjoy each other's company and have learned to understand and fulfill each other's emotional and physical needs. This is not easy, and should not be pursued if you are not ready to live with the consequences of your decision. Don't rush, having the right person is important and you should take the time to ensure your mate selection will produce harmony in your life. The pain associated with a dysfunctional relationship and divorce requires that we give this decision all the seriousness it deserves.

Divorce, Remarry? Never Again, so We Thought!

What about those who were married and are now divorced? Is there life after divorce? The answer is yes! But first, you need to go back to the "start" and reevaluate why you failed the first time around. Some people will say you need at least five years to get healthy; I don't know what the magic number is, because it depends on you and your personal history or emotional seabag, but I do believe that weeks after your divorce was finalized is too soon! It is estimated that 60% of second marriages fail. One reason why they fail is the "empty bed" syndrome, which results in the development of room 1 to room 4 relationships.

Another reason why second marriages fail, is when the marriage is for primarily for economic security, which usually results in shallow relationships that don't last or are very unfulfilling. Giving credence to why—"If it at first you don't succeed try, try, try again"—does not apply to marital relationships. I had an associate who divorced, remarried, divorced and then remarried his original wife! "Is he happy?" is what you are probably asking yourselves, and for him the answer was no, and he divorced the first wife a second time! Marriage is not for the feeble hearted. Remarriage is tough and should be considered more critically than a first marriage. The emotional injury and financial losses to you and your marital partner requires you to carefully consider the ramifications of your decision to remarry, especially if you have children from the previous marriage.

Children and Remarriage

Divorce is tough on all parties concerned and affects a child's emotional development. Bottom line is if you have children and you remarry, your children are looking to you to be a good role model. Additionally, children may have the fantasy that their parents will remarry so they don't have to choose between their parents. If you remarry and you do not achieve harmony or oneness with your new spouse, your children will again be scarred and may face challenges obtaining and maintaining healthy relationships. If you succeed at remarriage, it could have a positive influence on your children's ideal of monogamy and contribute to their ability to develop into emotionally healthy adults.

I believe if you are a parent, your primary focus should be on that role even if it means delaying serious relationships until after your children have left the home. Unfortunately, some make the decision to remarry because of economic reasons. You can't neglect your responsibility to provide for your children's emotional stability, health, and physical safety. If the person you are involved with is not someone you would trust raising your children in the event that you suffered a debilitating illness or death, then the relationship should not be pursued. You should wait until you know your relationship is firmly in room 3 before introducing someone else to your children. This should allow you to know whether or not you would want this person to have any influence on your children and whether or not you are willing to make a long-term commitment to this person. Remember the law of the harvest when considering your relationships. It is helpful to look back once in a while to ensure you are plowing a field that has straight troughs and plants has that are worthy of harvesting.

Emotional and Financial Responsibility to Children

As I stated in the previous paragraph divorce is hard, especially on children. What makes that transition from having two parents to one even tougher is economic hardship. After a divorce, household income, on an average, experiences a 30% decrease. Regardless of the relationship you have with your children's parent, you have a responsibility to ensure your children have a safe place to live, access to adequate education, food, clothing, health care, and the other essentials that contribute to their quality of life. I know some people (primarily men) who justify not paying child support because they think their ex-spouse will monetarily benefit from their contribution and feel that is unacceptable. If your former spouse's quality of life improved because you paid your child support payments on time and regularly, your children's quality of life improves too. Like it or not, if the caregiver of your children has physical custody of your children, and along with you are co-contributors to your children's relationship needs accounts. Your decision not to contribute financially is equally as detrimental as your decision not to contribute to your children's relationship needs accounts.

I hope that after reading about the five relationship needs (love, acceptance, appreciation, respect, and trust) you realize the importance of establishing and maintaining your relationships with your children. Often, when the marital relationship ends, some parents forsake the relationship they have with their children. A large number of children living in divorced households do not have regular contact with the parent who no longer resides in the household. When a person chooses their relationship with a boyfriend or girlfriend over their relationship with their children, they are making a big mistake. You have a lifelong obligation to provide for your children's emotional and physical needs.

Sad but true story. An associate of mine ended up with the full custody of his son due to the incarceration of his ex-wife. Unfortunately, his second marriage was not harmonious and as such, he spent little to no time at home. This meant his new wife was the primary caregiver of his adolescent son. The results were tragic and his son was immersed into an environment of verbal berating and sometimes physical abuse from his stepmother. He also experienced physical and verbal abuse from his father. His life became a living hell in which he had no escape and he eventually ended up in a juvenile ward. His son's childhood experiences of an abusive stepmother and father were almost a mirror image of his own. Chances are his son will leave home, like him with inadequately filled relationship needs accounts and have difficult times sorting things out during the Separation phase of life (if he gets that far). Bottom line, do not neglect your children's emotional and financial needs. The consequences of your decision not to provide adequate emotional and financial support will affect on your children's ability to function normally as adults.

Work and Relationships

My father shared with me a phrase that has stuck with me for decades and that is "Don't get your money and honey in the same place." He told me that if you chose to have a relationship with a co-worker, it could have some detrimental consequences, especially if there are work policies that prohibit dating between co-workers. Your place of employment is where you spend the majority of your conscience time and a disharmonious relationship will be detrimental to your success at work and home. As stated earlier, we don't know where we will find love, and if you have found love in your place of employment, you need to think through the consequences of that decision, especially if you both have consensually agree to advance from room 2 to room 4.

Final Thoughts on Relationships

Finding a relationship that provides contentment and emotional support in this seemingly dog eat dog world can never be undervalued. I believe emotionally and financially stable men and women can achieve a joy that is beyond mere words. Finding the right person begins with you, because your mate is a reflection of you. If you want the best life has to offer then, you need to have respect for people and their ability to influence and or inspire you when the world seems without form and purpose. To modify the quote by Jeanne Mayo, "Show me your friends and I will show you your future," to say "Show me your spouse and I will show you your future," should clearly state why the decision to marry should not be taken lightly. Once you have identified with yourself and resolved whatever was placed in your Preparation phase emotional seabag, then you're ready to make one of the most important decisions you will ever make in your life and that is who should I marry. The "who you marry" question cannot be trivialized and requires maturity to approach it with the respect, reverence, and the sincerity it deserves.

Chapter 3

Room 4
How Do You Obtain Joy?

In the "relationship house" room 4 is where sexual activities occur. Introducing sex to a relationship may or may not improve the relationship. Joyful sexually encounters require consensual and mutual emotional and physical commitments. Because joyful sexual encounters are vital to the longevity of room 4 relationships, I have devoted a chapter to room 4.

I'd like to start out with two questions and answers. Is sex love? No! Is love sex? No! Sex and love are not interchangeable. Sex is not love, but it is normally confused with love. Some people think the act of sexual intercourse automatically establishes the joint five relationship needs accounts which couldn't be further from the truth. And love is not a prerequisite for sexual intercourse. If that were true, then sexual intercourse between strangers or casual acquaintances would never occur. A healthy sexual relationship is consensually giving of oneself to another person during the act of sexual intercourse. If sex is not consensual, then it is rape or some form of dominance and will not result in a mutually-gratifying experience! If you want to have joy in room four and maintain your self-respect, you should not give of yourself if there are not firmly established relationship needs accounts with the other person. Sex is also the physical act that creates life. I believe you should not share one of life's most precious gifts and responsibilities, the act that could create a child, if you do not have or desire to maintain a committed relationship.

Going back to the relationship house analogy, for those who did not progress through the house (in other words, consensually transitioned from room 1, 2, 3, and 4), the ability to have a lifelong joyful sexual relationship with their spouse may or may not occur. Instead of being a fulfilling aspect of the marital relationship, that can strengthen a couple's bond, it could be a source of disappointment and frustration. Understanding the physical differences between men and women can help to relieve some of the disappointments and frustrations that can exist in a physical relationship.

For starters, men and women are typically sexually aroused differently. Men are primarily stimulated by visual attraction, which alone can be enough to cause physical arousal. Most women require more than visual attraction. A woman might be visually attracted to a man, but she is not normally sexually aroused by his appearance alone. Additionally, most women will not respond to physical stimulation if she cannot connect with her emotions. Which gives credence to "men will play at love for sex and women will play at sex for love." Some women even go to the extent of faking sexual satisfaction in order to fulfill their need for love.

Therefore, men and women should have strong communication skills and, learn about each other's emotional and physical needs and have an understanding of human anatomy before engaging in sexual relationships. In an unhealthy, polygamous relationship, sex presents potential emotional and/or health risks. I recommend reserving sex for marriage or a long-term monogamous relationship, in other words, room 4 relationships. The confidence that comes from knowing you are in a committed and safe relationship, should create the conditions that would allow you to increase your sexual awareness without the fear of rejection or subjection to avoidable health risks.

Developing a Healthy Room Four Attitude

You have probably heard it by now, that the quality you will experience in whatever you pursue in life has a lot to do with your attitude. This is true about sex and the attitude you and your spouse have about sex will contribute to the desire to learn how to communicate each other's emotional and physical needs as well as each other's anatomy. If you think that good sex in marriage will just happen naturally, you're being naive! I know of men and women who even after being married and having children never achieved joy in their sex life. The reason why they did not achieve mutually satisfying experiences was different for each of them, but basically had to do with misguided attitudes about sex, and/or the couple's inability to maintain their five relationship needs accounts coupled with ignorance, insensitivity, and/or selfishness.

In order to have a healthy attitude about sex, it is important to know that sex in a committed monogamous and/or marital relationship is expected to be guilt free. Secondly, when you marry, both people should surrender themselves to a life of service, which is based on selfless giving. Willful submission to another person in a mutually reciprocating relationship is not being a doormat or sex toy. Marriage should be an atmosphere where both people are committed to outdoing each other in their ability to give selflessly without conditions and dominance in all aspects of the relationship, including sex. Both should be committed to making deposits in the joint relationship needs accounts without the expectation of making immediate withdrawals.

When you have two people who are committed to bringing joy to one another and encouraging each other, you have a relationship that will allow each person to be sensitive to their spouse's emotional and physical needs, which includes setting aside time for intimacy, sexual arousal and mutual contentment. Unfortunately, misconceptions about sex, can influence a couple's ability to develop the proper attitude toward sex. I am convinced that when God created mankind, joyous monogamous sexual relationships were in mind. Attitudes about sex have been distorted and have caused some to think that a blissful marital sexual relationship was in direct conflict with spiritual purity. Some cultures even go to the extreme of female genital mutilation to assure that sex is not mutually satisfying! Nothing could be further from the truth, if sex is within a monogamous marital relationship! Unless both the husband and wife develop the attitude that sex within marriage is healthy, then you will never achieve mutual sexual satisfaction in marriage. Some attitudes about sex are distorted by premarital sexual experiences that were damaging and did little to foster healthy attitudes about sex.

Some people may require counseling to overcome their preconceived notions about sex. Premarital counseling can allow a couple to understand the role of sex within marriage and identify potential barriers to a couple's ability to have a healthy marital sex life. For some men and women, a hormonal imbalance may affect their sex drive, which means consulting with a physician for possible medical treatment. The best medical treatment may have reduced effectiveness if you don't have a healthy attitude about marital sex. Mutually satisfying marital sex contributes to a lifelong fulfilling relationship because sex is an exclusive form of communication that binds a couple and contributes to a couple's sense of belonging.

Obstacles to Sexual Joy

Ignorance, insensitivity, and selfishness are obstacles that can prevent sexual joy. I believe if more men and women knew how powerful their compassion and sensitivity toward each other was to improving sexual prowess, more people would be cautious about their use of words. Case in point, a female coworker of mine openly discussed her marital congenital encounters during social gatherings. She often said her sexual encounters with her husband never lasted more than five minutes. To make matters even worse, she often compared her second husband's sexual performance to her first husband's prowess. It made people think to themselves, What's wrong with him? And why is she sharing this with us? It's a shame her lack of sensitivity resulted in public humiliation of her husband. Her reckless use of words eventually resulted in the death of their marriage. After their divorce, he remarried and was able to achieve a mutually gratifying relationship with a compassionate woman. What occurs in your bedroom is between you and your spouse, regardless of how persistent co-workers or friends may inquire. Unfortunately, the solution to their sexual dissatisfaction required openness to marital counseling, open communication and a commitment to resolving the issue, something my coworker desperately lacked.

In order to create and maintain an atmosphere of intimacy and remove the obstacles to sexual joy, requires mutual compassion and respect. When both people make earnest efforts to accept and understand each other and are committed to satisfying each other, it contributes to the couple's ability to achieve and sustain sexual joy.

Infidelity can destroy your sex life, presents a severe obstacle to sexual joy and empties the "trust" account. Sex results in the exchange of bodily fluids and should not be outside of a monogamous relationship. If you both practice monogamy, then genital secretions should not be a concern, but if you suspect your mate is not practicing fidelity, then you should be cautious and abstain until you know whether or not you are in a monogamous relationship. The use of condoms may reduce exposure to some genital secretions, but you are still subjecting yourselves to risks. Possible exposure to sexually transmitted diseases is just one of the reasons why you should reserve all forms of sex for marriage. It is the responsibility of both sexual partners to ensure they are free of sexually transmitted diseases and if you were involved in previous premarital sexual relationships, as a precaution, each of you should be medically evaluated to ensure you do not transmit a disease to your future marital partner.

Birth Control and Children

Another obstacle for couples that have decided to delay child bearing is having an effective and reliable birth control plan. Once you have made the decision to be sexually active, you must have a birth control plan and this advice applies to both genders. Being sexually active without a birth control plan is reckless and not only affects on you, but your sexual partner and your other relationships. Both partners are equally responsible for birth control. Because of the risk of pregnancy, I further warn females, that the decision to be sexually active has consequences that will remain with you for the rest of your life. Your responsibilities as a parent don't end when your child is age eighteen, you have the responsibilities of being a parent for the rest of your life! Since it takes two to tango, the warning also extends to men. If you are having unprotected sex, you are setting yourself up for sexual transmitted diseases, financial loss, and fathering children out of wedlock. Responsible men assure they use a condom to minimize the risks to themselves and their partner. Any man can father a child; it takes a real man to provide for a child's emotional, financial, and physical needs. This is almost impossible to do if your children are living in multiple households! Raising a child outside of a stable relationship is difficult and has financial obligations that exceed late Preparation or early Separation phase earning abilities. In a marriage or a long-term monogamous relationship, if either of you has a genuine fear of pregnancy, it will stymie intimacy.

Children need your emotional and financial support. Developing a plan and implementing it with your sexual partner, will help reduce or eliminate the fear of pregnancy. Caution: Implementation of a plan has to occur before you become sexually active, because a pregnancy can occur during your first sexual encounter. For married couples, if age is not a factor, I recommend waiting two to three years before having children. This will give your relationship time to develop the deep roots needed to sustain your marriage during the early child rearing years. Children have emotional and physical needs that require the couple to make sacrifices of their time and other resources.

Most women go through emotional and ALL will go through physical changes related to pregnancy and childbirth. I believe it is best to have the loving support of a spouse during this time of transformation. I also believe that one of the times when a woman is most radiant is when she is pregnant. A woman's radiance during pregnancy is stunning and if in a committed martial relationship, she should have the emotional, financial and physical support to have a memorable pregnancy. The emotional and physiological demands are more tolerable when you know there is someone who will be there beside you during your time of need.

Pregnancy and parenting of a newborn is demanding. The time commitment can be draining even when there are two people provid-ing for the needs of the newborn and can stymie a couple's intimacy. If you had many (and I do suggest numerous) happy pre-child rearing phase marital memories, it can help you regain that intimacy that may have been disrupted during the early stages of parenting.

Key to Intimacy—Relaxation

Ever wondered why the marriage ceremony should be followed by a honeymoon? The honeymoon is supposed to be the couple's time away from day to day activities (to include social media) and give the new couple an opportunity to relax and enjoy their new beginning. The key to success in your sexual relationship is teaching each other about what "turns me on" and "what brings you joy" in your lifelong journey, which ideally should begin during the honeymoon. If faced with cutting wedding expenses, don't sacrifice the honeymoon for a bigger reception because receptions don't build long-term intimacy! Couples with healthy sex lives are people who are confident and empowered! Men and women need to communicate their desires and needs to their lover and set-aside time for relaxation and intimacy. If you don't set boundaries for intimacy, such as establishing a date night or other exclusive relaxation time, the business of live will easily encroach and suffocate intimacy.

Pleasure versus Joy

I don't know if you have picked up on it, but when I have described the feeling you get from a room 4 relationship, I used the word "joy" instead of "pleasure." Pleasure is engagement in activity that brings about temporary happiness and is usually followed by guilt. Additionally, pleasurable activities are normally motivated by selfishness and are without regard to the other person's desires or needs. Pleasurable activities temporarily stimulate your senses and in the long run require increased levels of stimulation to reach that same feeling you had before. This need for increased level of stimulation, is what leads to addictive behavior and eventually robs you of any feeling of long-term contentment. Joy comes from an internal source of contentment, regardless of your environment and is not because of selfish desires, but from giving. Joy in a room 4 relationship, is when two people share their internal contentment to create an environ-ment of fulfillment and satisfaction. Unfortunately, modern culture (art, films, magazines, and music) does little to discourage engage-ment in selfish activities, because vulgarity is profitable and self-discipline is considered to be prudish and unprofitable.

Final Thoughts on Room 4

I want to warn you about the dangers of seeking pleasures because it can eventually lead to the development of destructive habits. Prevention is far better than taking corrective action, because old habits are hard to break. By avoiding non-emotional, non-monogamous sexual activities, you are exercising preventative measures that will save you from suffering severe losses.

Lastly, I personally believe nothing is more gratifying than a blissful marital relationship. Fruits of joyful marital relationships are happy families and the confidence a person needs to pursue their dreams and goals. Maintaining fidelity will result in years of guilt-free room 4 expressions of love and joy

Chapter 4

Money
Steward or Squander?

Almost every child dreams of having enough money to go to the store and buy all the toys they ever wanted, or to buy ice-cream for all their friends on a hot summer's day. What's wrong with wanting money? It depends on what value you have placed on money. Is it a tool that you use as a faithful steward or is it something you desire regardless of the moral or physical costs? The answer to the previous question will determine if money has the proper perspective in your life. You are probably asking yourself, how much money is enough? It depends on how you answered the previous question. If you answered, "As a tool of a faithful and good steward," then you will probably learn to live below your means (and living below your means doesn't mean living in poverty!) A steward is a caretaker of property and understands whatever they accumulate here on earth (there are no trailers behind hearses!) will one day transfer to someone else.

If you are a steward, you recognize that you have a responsibility to ensure the resources that are under your care are properly managed and higher principles guide your decisions. If you answered, "Desire regardless of cost," then you will probably never have enough because you are acting as the final owner who can recklessly dispose of the resource and believe you are not accountable to anyone. If you make $250,000 (USD) a year in the year 2023 or its equivalent in the future, most will say you have good income. I would agree, but if you earn $250,000 a year and spend $249,995 a year with no savings, then you are poor! If you can't learn to live below your means, then it does not matter if you make $40,000 or $5,000,000 a year you will never have enough.

Putting Money into Its Proper Perspective

The value people place on money is often developed during the Preparation phase of life. Children whose parents or role models put money into its proper perspective and taught them the value of knowing the difference between "needs and wants" will generally learn how to live below their means. The ability to discern between "needs and wants" allows you to have the discipline to tell yourself "no" and provides you the ability to save regardless of how meager your salary may be because you will find a way to live below your means. As Sheryl Crow, wrote so eloquently in her song "Soak up the Sun," "It's not having what you want, it's wanting what we got." This kind of attitude will contribute to your ability to live within your means and not letting your wants drive you to financial ruin.

If you want to be a successful steward, you have to learn how to manage and respect the items of little value before you are trusted with high-valued assets. Who would trust anyone with a million-dollar project, if they grossly mismanaged a twenty-thousand-dollar project? The answer is no one! Don't get the illusion that having more money will automatically make you a better manager. All you have to do is look at the number of lottery winners who later became broke because of mismanagement of their money. Many people desire to be rich and young and I'd like to remind people of the quote by Mark Twain, "Youth is wonderful. It's a shame to waste it on the young."

Acquiring wealth when you are immature (no age limit here, you can be forty years old and still be immature!) is like giving a loaded semiautomatic pistol to a three-year-old! Without intervention, the results will be tragic for all those involved! Without discipline and maturity, the resources would be wasted and would be the equivalent of giving a toddler a full glass of red wine and asking them to walk across your white carpet and give the glass to your mate.

By time they get there (if ever), your wine would be gone and your carpet destroyed! If you want to be financial independent, you need to exercise self-discipline and be prepared to run the race you can't afford to lose. The race against time is one that no one can afford to lose, because time doesn't grant any special privileges to anyone and is nonrefundable.

The Race You Can't Afford to Lose

Each person that lives (oh, by the way, tomorrow is not promised to anyone!) starts the day with the opportunity to use twenty-four hours or 86,400 seconds a day and what you do with it makes a big difference on the rate of return. Are you getting the best rate of return on your time investment? To answer that question, you need to ask yourself what do you do with your time and what are you doing to prepare for the future? For example, if you are in the Separation phase of life and you are attending college, a trade school, or working as an apprentice, then you are hoping your time and financial (yours and/or your parents!) investments will pay off in future higher salaries. Having a college degree or advanced technical training is no guarantee of higher salaries, but it significantly increases your possibilities. I believe completion of an educational goal improves an individual's level of self-confidence. What a college degree or completion of technical training says to your future employer, is that you have the self-discipline needed to start and complete an educational goal and you are trainable. Companies are reluctant to take their hard-earned capital and invest into someone who has not demonstrated their ability to start and finish an educational goal. I also believe your grade point average (GPA) states how well you can focus your mind to the completion of your educational goal.

As I stated earlier, having a college degree or technical training does not guarantee higher salaries, and if it doesn't then you have to ask yourself what does? You need to have a vision of where you want to be and an unstoppable desire to achieve it! Helen Keller was once asked if there was anything worse than losing one's sight.

She responded, "Yes, losing one's vision."

You need to have a vision about your future. If you haven't defined your vision, then it is time to start working on it. A person without vision is like a car with no gas or a boat without a rudder. In other words, you can be physically and mentally healthy, but if you lack personal drive, initiative, and a personal vision, you are not going to achieve more than mediocre performance. Your vision can drive you and inspire you to have the self-discipline you will need to help you build the good habits you need to achieve your goals.

Learning about Money

What do you do with money once you start trading your time for it (and, oh by the way, you started trading time for money the day you started your first job)? First, you need to realize that you are only a steward of the money that you are earning. Secondly, retirement is not a matter of age, but whether or not you have enough passive income to support your standard of living without working, in other words, financially independent. And you don't have to be old and gray to be financially independent! Thirdly, you need to have a realistic budget based on needs not wants, that is, if you don't want to live paycheck to paycheck for the rest of your life! If you develop a budget, you need to account for the need to have savings to create and maintain an emergency fund, in other words, pay yourself first! An emergency fund is three to six months of your household expenses that can be used in the event that you are unable to trade your time for money.

Buy Now, Pay Later—Charge It (Not)!

No discussion about money would be complete without a discussion about credit. The ability to gain information about you has never been easier and is one of the reasons why identity theft is one of the fastest growing crimes! Your credit history is a permanent record that never goes away. Your ability to manage your credit is important to reducing the costs associated with borrowing money, car insurance premiums, and even your ability to get job, rent an apartment, or buy a house. Creditors, future employers, and insurers use your credit score to determine if you are trustworthy and to assess their risk in establishing a relationship with you! Whether or not you agree with this, it does not take away the need to understand why credit is important. With self-discipline and monitoring, you can assure your credit history is an asset and not a liability. Most people in the early Separation phase of life, provided their parents or siblings did not use their identity (yes, family members abuse each other's personal information to establish credit), you probably have no credit score at all because you have no credit history.

Several factors contribute to your credit score, but I have found three factors that have a great affect on your credit score: payment history, credit-to-debt ratio, and length of credit. When you establish a line of credit, credit card, student loan, auto loan, personal line of credit, etc., the company you make payments to reports to one or all three the major credit bureaus, Equifax (Beacon), Experian (FICO), or TransUnion. Your credit score can range from a low of 300 to a high of 850, dependent on the scoring model used by the credit bureau. The credit bureau(s) receive the report on how you did that month. Were you on time or were you late? If you were late for more than thirty days, that goes on your credit report and is a mark against your credit score. The longer you take to bring your account to current, the greater the damage to your credit score. Because of the costs associated with reporting, most creditors report your account status once a month, so it may take sixty days before corrective action is reflected on the credit report and associated credit score.

Another factor influencing your credit score is credit-to-debt ratio. Credit-to-debt ratio is the ratio of your debt to your approved line of credit. If your credit card has a $1,000 credit limit and your balance is $900, you have an unhealthy credit-to-debt ratio of 90 % ($900/$1000 = .90). This affects your credit score, even if you make your payments on time. Your balance begins to have less influence on your credit score when it is below 70% of your credit limit. I recommend that you don't maintain a balance on your credit card because of the costs associated with using someone else's money. If you are trying to establish credit, it may be necessary to carry low a balance, but I recommend that you keep the balance below 25% and pay it off after six months.

The third factor contributing your credit score is length of credit. How long you have had a credit line, can also factor into your credit score. The creditors want to know how you did over a period of time. If you don't have any payment history that is longer than six months, it does little to show how you will do with a major purchase that may require you to make payments for thirty-six months or thirty years (typical home mortgage).

With those kinds of consequences and time commitment, you may be asking yourself, "Why do I need credit?" Good question, one that is worthy of your understanding and respect. Sensible people reserve the use of credit for the purchase of high-priced items and not extending their paycheck! For example, most people don't have $500,000 to purchase a home in their savings account! Having an established credit history allows you to borrow the money you need for a major purchase at a reasonable interest rate. Other major purchases like a car normally exceed most people's discretionary funds. Even if you have thirty thousand dollars to purchase a vehicle, smart investors would rather let their assets grow (compounded interest is optimized when you have more principle) instead of spending it on something that depreciates immediately after you sign the transfer of ownership documents! This is especially true if the rate of return on their investments has the potential to exceed the loan interest rate.

Credit, like money, is a tool, but it can be detrimental if not used properly. When your debt payments prevent you from having a savings program, then you are in trouble. Credit is just one more reason why you need to be able to tell yourself "No" and why you have to develop a needs-versus-wants attitude about spending. This also applies to student loans. It could be tempting to borrow more than you need and before you know it, the repayment of the student loans will impact on your ability to pursue your other long-term financial goals. I do recommend that you pursue establishing credit gradually before you attempt to establish your personal residence away from your family during the Separation phase of life. You can establish credit, even if you don't have any credit history, in other words, your credit score is zero or not applicable. Your first line of credit will usually be based on other factors, such as your ability to repay the debt, in other words a stable job, a cosigner and/or how you managed your accounts at financial institutions. If you have savings and/or a checking account and did not overdraw your account (due recklessness behavior), then your bank or credit union could be your first source of credit. You can also do this by obtaining a store credit card to pay for a purchase (I suggest a purchase between three hundred and five hundred dollars) and pay it off over a six-month period of time.

Once you have established a credit profile, you should be able to obtain a credit card. Caution: Having a cosigner is placing your debt obligation on someone else. The cosigner's credit history and income are being used along with your information to determine if the loan or line of credit will be approved. If you do not pay on time, it hurts your credit history and cosigner's and the creditor can force the cosigner to repay the debt. I do not recommend having a cosigner for a credit card and this should only be for a debt obligation that has a fixed and not an indefinite term. The shorter the better. If you need a cosigner to establish credit, I recommend that you don't obligate the cosigner to a loan for longer than twenty-four months. I have seen cosigning agreements totally destroy relationships and this should not be taken lightly and fall in the trust but verify category. If you decide to have a cosigner, I recommend the statements be sent to the cosigner's address. This will assure the cosigner is aware of the status of the financial obligation. The statements also allow the cosigner to know if you are current and provide the ability to intervene, if necessary, to avoid damage to their credit history and score. If you are having problems, contact the cosigner and work out a plan to get on track. No one likes unpleasant surprises! Cosigner relationships should never be with friends or coworkers and I do not recommend that you go outside the boundaries of your immediate family, which may need to include a grandparent (some parents have poor credit history!), to find a cosigner.

If you keep in mind the three factors that influence your credit score, (payment history, credit-to-debt ratio, and length of credit) you can be on your way to building a reputable credit profile. Even if you have blown your credit history and scores because of previous reckless behavior, you can apply these principles to improve your credit scores; just remember those past mistakes don't go away and will require a commitment to responsible use of credit to diminish their affect on your credit score. This analogy maybe helpful, you can view your credit score like a class grade. If you started the semester with a 2.0, it is going to take a lot of A's to bring your grade to 3.5 or higher and we all know this doesn't happen overnight and requires a lot of hard work and dedication!

Budget Basics

A budget can be used to help you develop a needs-versus-wants attitude and help you manage credit. Having a budget allows you to manage your expenses and can provide you with the tools necessary to manage your debts. The financial industry recommends your consumer debt, less housing expenses, be less than 20% of your "after-deductions pay" also known as "net" or "after-tax pay." Caution: Don't base your debt ratio on your credit cards' minimum payments and think that everything is okay! If you only pay the minimum, you will always be in debt and would overpay five or more times your purchases made using credit (imagine a hundred-dollar-Big Mac!) Ideally, you should always want to be as close to zero as possible because when you are debt-free, you are truly free. For example, your net monthly pay is $3,500, then your maximum debt payment should be less than $700 per month ($700/$3,500 = 20%) and this includes the costs of vehicle financing.

Life Insurance Basics

Why do you need life insurance? Because no one gets out alive and during life we are all subjected to health hazards! Sooner or later, we will ALL die and no one knows the exact day, month, year, or hour of their death. Therefore, it is important to have a basic understanding of why you need life insurance. Insurance allows people to share loses by pooling their resources with others. Therefore, the insurance company is not nameless or faceless, it's me and you! In the event of a loss, assets are taken from those who shared the risk at the time of loss. Life insurance provides payment to your beneficiaries after your death and can allow them to have the financial resources to pay for your funeral. Life insurance can provide your beneficiaries the ability to pay off or pay down your liabilities, such as credit cards, car and/or education loans and other financial commitments.

There are many different types of group and individual life insurance policies, but typically the insurance company will require you to be in relatively good health. Your arrest record, health, and driving record may determine whether or not you can be insured. In the case of life insurance, your age, gender, health and tobacco usage are other factors affecting the cost of life insurance. A steward plans for the worst, while hoping for the best, and having life insurance is a prudent way to prepare for the worst.

Cars—How Fast, How Much?

I have yet to go to a corner of the world and not see someone who doesn't admire a beautiful car, and this is true for both genders. Instead of cars being used a tool to get us to and from work or provide us the ability run errands or other transportation needs, they sometimes become inordinate liabilities instead of reasonably acquired resources. Men are especially susceptible to visual stimulants and as such are naturally drawn to beautiful cars.

For some, a car can be an unhealthy obsession. Allowing a car to become an unhealthy obsession can result in financial ruin. Since a car is a tool and has no other intrinsic purpose, other than possibly propping up low self-esteem, you should limit yourself to only buying a car that you can afford. If you dedicate a large percentage of your income to acquiring, insuring and maintaining a car, (it is advisable to keep all debt payments to 20% or less of your net income) then you will be hard pressed to have sufficient income for housing, charitable contributions, savings, living expenses such as food and clothing and remaining discretionary income (i.e., entertainment).

A fact a lot of young people overlook when they are looking for a car is cost of insurance and maintenance. Because of the need to control the cost of maintenance, I recommend a low-cost entry-level new or slightly-used vehicle that has a manufacturer's warranty over a comparably priced used luxury model that does not have a manufacturer's warranty. If you did not take the time to investigate the costs associated with insuring and maintaining the vehicle, you could be setting yourself up for financial disappointment and frustration. What good is having a car and no discretionary income? If the person you are attracted to is only interested in you because of the car you drive, then you can expect their other interests in you to be shallow. Also, it doesn't make sense to spend four thousand dollars accessorizing a $1,500-car and the results are usually ridiculous.

Remember, a car is not a financial investment! In fact, for a car to be a financial investment, it would have to be a collector's item that few people can afford. Even when purchased new, it suddenly depreciates by as much as 5% after it changes status from new to used vehicle, which happens once the car is registered to its new owner! And the transfer of ownership happens before you leave the dealership (remember the paperwork you signed!) If you are considering a new or used vehicle, do your research! Find out how much the car is worth based on its features by checking with your local financial institution or the Internet. If you are purchasing a used car, take the car to an independent dealer that routinely services that brand of vehicle. There will be an expense related to this inspection, but having the used car inspected by a facility that routinely services that brand of vehicle, can possibly identify malfunctions that could result in huge financial liabilities shortly after the acquisition of the vehicle.

It also helps to develop the right attitude about vehicle acquisition. In other words, don't fall in love with the vehicle; just like the relationship house, when you emotionally commit too early, you are setting yourself up for failure. If the vehicle acquisition costs (down payment, plus monthly payments), insurance, corrective and preventive maintenance costs don't meet acceptable standards, then the lack of emotional commitment will allow you to gracefully walk away. Lack of emotional commitment will reduce your vulnerability to unorthodox sales practices. Bottom line, a car is a tool that can provide you with freedom of mobility, but if not pursued with the proper attitude and perspective, it can result in years of unrealistic financial obligations that will act as chains and restrict your financial and personal mobility.

Career Choices

Developing a relentless desire to achieve your vision is vital to running a competitive pace in the marathon called life. What does "possess a relentless desire to achieve a vision" have to do with career choices? I have discovered during my life's journey, that people like predictability and structure and most will sacrifice a chance for an opportunity for security (remember Maslow's needs hierarchy?) Most people hate change and are afraid of it and it shows in their personal choices. If you are in a dead-end job that barely meets your needs or the needs of a family, then it is time to use your burning desire and embrace some risks.

Case in point, I started out my employment career at age thirteen by working as a school janitor. I eventually graduated from high school and enlisted in the US Navy. After being in the military for a year and coming home on leave, I was surprised by colleagues who adjusted their lifestyle to the wages they earned from employment as a part-time janitor. Some of them were comfortable and afraid of risk. Eventually, they had to change because the income was too meager to support their needs in the Separation phase of life. Let's be clear, I am not looking down on anyone who has an entry-level job. Just assure your aspirations are set higher so you don't limit yourself to greater opportunities. If you don't have a vision that is morally aligned, then you could be setting yourself up for years of frustration.

If the career you desire requires education or training, then take a chance and enroll yourself into an institution that can provide you with the skills you need to achieve your goals. The sooner, the better! If you followed the principles I stated earlier in "Getting First Things First," then you should have low levels of responsibilities and the ability to focus on obtaining the skills you need or want to possess. I am not saying if you are married with children that you should not take calculated risks to achieve your life's desire, but you can't ignore your responsibilities to your family.

Another reason why your career choice is important is because if you are performing an occupation that is compatible with your personality, then your chances of being successful are immensely improved. If you don't know what type of occupation suits you, then I recommend you take advantage of a career assessment. There may be occupations you never even considered because you were not exposed to them. I would not wish the drudgery of performing a job you don't like on anyone, regardless of how much they are paid! Most people spend the majority of their conscious hours at work and if you are miserable because you hate your occupation, then most of your time is filled with dissatisfaction. Don't think I am trying to place a higher value to work than relationships, but if you are working and don't like what you do, your labor is emotionally and physically draining. This is not giving you an excuse to sit around and do nothing, but if you have prepared yourself and you are committed to your vision, you will have to spend some time in the trenches, but your hard work and vision should allow you to elevate yourself to the reach the stars.

Are You an Entrepreneur?

If your occupation doesn't provide the independence to create your own personal "niche" and that is more important to you than supporting the company or organization you are trading your time for wages, then it might be time to consider going into business for yourself. Every state has a Small Business Administration (SBA) office. The SBA almost always has material on how to obtain financing for your business venture and/or low costs educational seminars to help you learn how to be your own boss. Most of the truly successful people in the world took their vision and shared it with others. Bill Gates dropped out of Harvard and starting his quest for his vision and look where he is now. Ray Kroc went from being a milkshake machine salesman, to a man who started a franchise called

McDonalds! Having a vision, coupled with a burning desire, has led to the creation of many of successful business ventures. Owning and operating a business is not without risk, but the highest rewards are normally set aside for those who are willing to take the biggest risks. Successful entrepreneurs do not let failure deter them from achieving their goals.

The definition of success has many different interpretations and what it is for you may be different from your neighbor or sibling. I encourage you to step outside your comfort zone, because those closest to you may be blocking your ability to see what's possible. Mark Twain said, "20 years from now you will be more disappointed about the things you did not do, instead the things you did wrong. So throw off your bow lines and set sail to achieve your heart's desire." Having a commitment coupled with a burning desire to achieve a noteworthy vision is important and can allow you to have a life that won't be riddled with regret. Having a vision doesn't guarantee success, but knowing you fought a good fight and ran a good race is more valuable than monetary gains alone.

The Financial Seasons (Spring, Summer, Fall, and Winter)

The four phases of life, Preparation, Separation, Independence, and Dependent, which have to do with your physical abilities, emotional development, and maturity, run parallel with the financial seasons of your life. We are born needing support (spring), separated and gain our independence (summer and fall), and when we are too old or unable to take care of ourselves and need to rely on the support of others and/or the assets we have acquired (winter).

A SAILOR'S ADVICE ON LIFE

Four Phases of Life

| Preparation (0 – 18?) | Separation (18 – 28?) | Independence (28 - ??) | Dependent (85 - ??) |

Financial Seasons

| Spring | Summer | Fall | Winter |

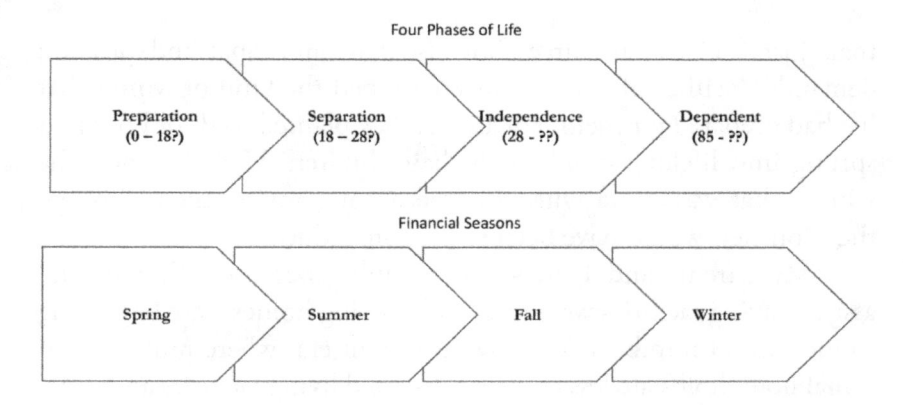

Figure 4 - 1

The quality of your life in the various seasons of life depends on whether or not those responsible for you during the Spring of your life were good stewards in the use of their resources of Love, Money and Time. If they were good stewards, then the probability of you becoming a good steward is significantly improved. If you are not a good steward of the resources you acquired in the Summer and early Fall of life, it will result into a cold and harsh winter. Respecting the law of the harvest is an important concept to understand when you are trying to leverage time as an ally. If you don't plant enough seeds, in other words invest your time and money wisely, then your harvest will be sparse when you are older. Some people have a "got to have it now" philosophy and this will normally guarantee a sparse harvest that will most likely be unable to meet their future needs. Moderation, regardless of your level of wealth, is the key to managing your resources.

Warning: What I presented was an ideal time line! Winter begins when you are no longer able to trade dollars for your time; your passive income cannot take care of you; and/or you can't physically or mentally take care of yourself (remember the Mark Twain youth quote?) As a baby boomer, I have journeyed with my parents during the winter season of their lives and have countless acquaintances, coworkers, and friends who have made or are on the journey with their sibling(s) or parent(s). The winter season requires more than just financial resources but also has emotional and physical demands. Neither of my parents envisioned the kind of winter that life had prepared for them. Fortunate, they planted seeds of Love that sprung into lifelong bonds with their children. Had they not, the winter, that was harsh with children accompanying them through their journey, would have been even more arduous.

My parents and I grew up in multigenerational homes and assisted living facilities were rare, and nursing homes were beginning to increase in numbers. We now live in an era, where multigenerational households are less common, assisted living facilities and nursing homes are experiencing a boom. These facilities have a coined the phrase "age in place" which basically means, if you can afford it, this is your final home. If you thought day care for young children was expensive, assisted living and skilled nursing homes have that beat hands down! If you want an idea of how expensive it could be, do an internet search on the "average cost of care" and if that glimpse into the costs of a winter season of life does not motivate you to plant good seeds, then I don't know what will!

If you don't have a family member in an assisted living facility, then I recommend you volunteer at a facility so you can have a first-hand look at what life is like in the winter season of life. If you do have a family member in a winter season of their life, I encourage you to spend some time with them since visitation rates are low at these facilities. Therefore, I encourage everyone to enjoy the season they are in! Just don't fall into the "got to have it now" syndrome so you can be the ant and not the grasshopper who did not prepare for the the winter!

Remember, it is not how much money you make, but how much of your money can you keep, which comes from learning to live well below your income. If you don't sacrifice some of your wants now, then you won't have enough money for the future. It does not take a lot of money to generate a sizable nest egg. The sooner you start living below your means, the better your chances to having a comfortable lifestyle during the late fall and winter seasons of life. If you have ever seen bumper sticker "We're spending our children's inheritance," then you have probably identified why selfishness contributes to poor savings habits.

When I first joined the Navy, one of my shipmate's parents chose to pay cash for a new sports car instead of helping their only child with her college education (remember what I said about cars not being financial investments and the winter season of life!) She eventually went to college after serving four years in the military, but their decision had a negative effect on their parent-to-child relationship. There is a proverb that says, "A good man leaves an inheritance for his children's children" (Proverbs 13:22).

Learning how to be financially responsible is very important and can determine whether or not your descendants are able to rise above mediocrity. Developing financial maturity takes time and it is reckless to provide wealth without guidance and restrictions to an immature recipient. There are enough examples of rich kids that have self-destructed from wealth received too early in life (remember the toddler with the glass of red wine?) In some cultures, where large families are the norm, the parents struggle to provide for the education of their oldest child and look to that child to assist in the financing of their siblings' education.

Once you realize that money is a tool and that you are only a steward, then your ability to leave a legacy worth having increases. Leaving a legacy is not just leaving behind financial assets, but it is also modeling and teaching your heirs how to be good stewards. If you ran your race pursuing goals worthy of your time and personal sacrifices, then you can expect a harvest that will be plentiful. Keeping "an end in mind" focus allows you to properly evaluate whether or not you will enjoy life in the late fall and winter seasons of life. Your burning desire to achieve a morally-responsible vision, can provide the fuel you need to keep running the race that will be worthy of recognition by your future generations. Financial independence is achievable, but requires the ability to live below your means and a desire to leave a legacy for generations to come.

I hope after reading the following words written by an anonymous writer, you will understand that we are just stewards during our journey called life.

"The Suitcase"
A man died...
When he realized it, he saw God coming closer with a suitcase in his hand.
Dialog between God and Dead Man
God: Alright son, it's time to go.
Man: So soon? I had a lot of plans...
God: I am sorry but, it's time to go.
Man: What do you have in that suitcase?
God: Your belongings.
Man: My belongings? You mean my things... Clothes... money...
God: Those things were never yours, they belong to the Earth.
Man: Is it my memories?
God: No. They belong to Time.
Man: Is it my talent?
God: No. They belong to Circumstance.
Man: Is it my friends and family?
God: No son. They belong to the Path you travelled.
Man: Is it my wife and children?
God: No. they belong to your Heart
Man: Then it must be my body!
God: No No... It belongs to Dust.
Man: Then surely it must be my Soul!
God: You are sadly mistaken son. Your Soul belongs to me.
Man with tears in his eyes and full of fear took the suitcase from the God's hand and opened it...
Empty! Heartbroken and tears running down his cheek, he asks God...
Man: I never owned anything?
God: That's Right. You never owned anything.

A SAILOR'S ADVICE ON LIFE

Man: Then? What was mine?
God: Your Moments. Every moment you lived was yours.
Life is just a Moment. Live it. Love it. Enjoy it.

Chapter 5

Starting and Finishing Strong

Decision-Making 101

Now that you have some understanding of what influences you as a person, I feel it is time to talk about your decision-making process. Unfortunately, some people spend more time reacting instead of responding to a set of circumstances. Don't get me wrong there are certain instances when a reaction is better than a response, such as removing your hand from a heat source! But unfortunately, more times than not, reacting (acting before thinking) can be very costly. First, you need to realize you have the freedom to choose your decisions, but you do not have the freedom to choose the consequences. For example, you can <u>choose</u> to cheat on your final exam, but if you are caught, you do not get to <u>choose</u> the consequences, such as expulsion from school or a failing a class. Using phrases such as "you made me mad" is irresponsible and reflects reacting instead of responding. How you handle anger, disappointment, and frustration is your choice and not someone else's! Maturity is realizing you have to accept the consequences of your decisions. The sooner you come to that conclusion, then the sooner you will begin to choose to respond vice react. Learning to think before you act will help you avoid a lot of calamity.

People are faced with choices that require them to consciously decide to either accept or reject participation in a potentially destructive behavior. Some critical decision-making "teething" occurs during the late Preparation and early Separation phases of life, in which a reverent spirit of rebellion is used to encourage you to put some distance between yourself and your parents and or guardians. For some, the rebellious acts are acceptable, such as choosing to tell your parents when you are sixteen and your family is planning their activities, that you are choosing to stay home instead of going with them to the movies. This desire for independence is healthy and most parents will recognize your need for independence, especially when you exhibit respect and self-control. Destructive rebellious acts, such as smoking marijuana, stealing your parents' money, and underage drinking are just a few examples of unacceptable behavior, and instead of gaining independence, it will cause rifts in your child-to-parent relationship due to violations of trust and or disrespectful attitudes due to excessive withdrawals from your parent(guardian)-to-child relationship needs accounts. You have a responsibility to make deposits to your five relationship needs accounts (love, acceptance, appreciation, respect, and trust) in all of your relationships and excessive withdrawals due to rebellious behavior will destroy the quality of those relationships!

Unfortunately, I know of too many "true life" stories of people who did not understand "decision-making 101." If you want the opportunity to see the consequences of bad decision making, spend some time in your local civil or criminal court as a member of the public. After listening to three or four cases, you will have an understanding of the consequences of bad decision making. Not everyone survives the consequences of their decisions. A young man I once knew was listening to his peers brag about the sex they were having with different women. He listened, but did not have anything to contribute because he was a twenty-year-old virgin. One night, he decided to change all that and paid a prostitute for sex. Unfortunately for him, in addition to losing his virginity, he contracted a venereal disease called "gonorrhea." Several weeks after he received treatment for gonorrhea, he was informed that he was also HIV-positive, the virus that causes AIDS. This was in 1993 and when contracting HIV was a death sentence. Imagine how he must have felt about his decision to engage in polygamous, unprotected sex. His decision to have sex with a prostitute and choosing not to use a condom would eventually result in his death.

Another young man decided he would show his friends how tough he was and chugged down a fifth of a bottle of whisky. This was after a whole day of drinking! Unfortunately, his act resulted in his death. He died from alcohol poisoning which caused him to suffer in the hospital for three days while he was literally fighting for his life. Can you imagine being the military supervisor who had to inform his family of his death; the family that had to live with the thought that their son's death was due to his own negligence; or the friends that could have stopped him from literally drinking himself to death?

If you think I am telling you these stories to scare you, you are right! Each of these acts took less than ten minutes for these people to carry out and the consequences affected them for the rest of their lives! Another factor that influenced both of these individuals' decision was their need to feel accepted by their peers. You need to think about your choices, because once you have decided and take action, it is like trying to do the impossible act of recalling a bullet from a fired weapon!

Using this analogy is healthy to understanding why your decision-making process is so important. Think of each of your decisions as seeds that you plant (some you will even forget you even planted!) that one day, you will have to harvest. Unfortunately, you do not get to choose whether or not you will harvest the seeds. The harvest will yield either healthy plants capable of bearing fruit and vegetables needed for growth and sustainment of life or be destructive weeds that stifle your healthy plants' growth. Don't get me wrong, everyone will plant some weeds, but a harvest full of weeds and no crops reflects habitual bad decision-making and will result in a miserable life.

Each decision we make, whether good or bad, requires critical resources, such as time (nonrefundable), finances, emotional, and health (your health is your wealth) investments. These resources will be used to either cultivate the growth of healthy plants or weeds. The choice is yours!

Faith and Its Impact on Decisions

All the previous thoughts I provided about decision-making focused on an individual's responsibility to make healthy decisions. I want to challenge you to consider how a belief system can have a positive influence on your ability to make healthy choices. The recognized major religions have a central theme and that is there are boundaries or guidelines to live by and acknowledgement there is an authority or an entity more powerful than mankind. The best definition of religion that I have heard is that religion is doing things that bring about positive changes in you (habits that bring about positive change). The desire to develop and maintain a positive relationship with God and the desire to willingly submit to a lifestyle that subscribes to self-denial in exchange for spiritual purity, has its merits and can assist you in developing the willpower or self-discipline necessary to avoid yielding to temptation. If you don't think a faith-based belief religion can have a positive influence on your life, then I challenge you to at least consider exploring your spirituality. Let's be clear—I am not recommending mind control or any belief that discriminates or is based on hate, but an opportunity to explore life with spiritual boundaries that guide your physical acts. If the religion you are practicing does not encourage you to improve the way you interact with humanity, then you need to consider a different spiritual journey.

Who Needs Guilt?

Some choices, in the beginning, seem harmless and may not seem to have any consequences. Unfortunately, when you engage in activities that you know you should not do and do not abstain from them, you are numbing yourselves to guilt. Guilt is that bad feeling you have when you do something wrong and can be a tool to help you develop good decision-making principles. If you have not realized the importance of recognizing a higher level of authority than yourself, then guilt should remind you that you are accountable for your decisions. Take if you will the following visual analogy to help you to understand the purpose of guilt in your decision-making. If you have ever operated an automobile, you notice certain warning lights like, check engine, oil, brakes, and other warning lights that come on when you switch your car's ignition switch to on. If the vehicle is operating normally, the warning lights will go off after you start the engine. When something goes wrong with the car, the warning lights are designed to get your attention and to tell you that something is wrong. Guilt works in the same way as the warning lights in your automobile. Guilt is used to warn you that something is wrong. Like your automobile, you can choose to ignore the warning light or you can have the car checked. If you choose to ignore the warning light, then you could suffer some tragic consequences, especially if the warning light was brakes or oil!

Most people who have a corrupted value system, don't become bad all at once. It is usually the result of a series of minor engagement in hidden unethical activities, that numbs their response to guilt. Nothing stays hidden forever, sooner or later it will come to light and you will have to face the consequences of your decisions (Remember the law of the harvest!) Unfortunately, most people don't take corrective action until they are required to suffer the consequences of their decisions. Bottom line, don't ignore guilt, use it as a way to avoid incrementally corrupting your value system.

Even if you had a pattern of bad decisions in the past, it is essential for you to learn that you don't have to keep making those choices. It is up to you to decide whether or not you will succeed or fail. Nothing is more heartbreaking than seeing a mentally and physically healthy man or woman destroy their life because of poor decision-making. I believe that understanding your weaknesses and vulnerabilities, coupled with acknowledging a higher level of authority, can make positive differences on your decision-making ability. This Bible verse has provided me comfort during my times of weakness. "And he said unto me, My grace is sufficient for thee: for my strength is made perfect in weakness." (2 Corinthians 12:9) Those who had horrible childhoods and inadequate relationship needs accounts, eventually discover that society, rightfully so, will hold them accountable for their choices. Our juvenile detention centers, jails, and prisons are full of people who are paying the price for their decisions. I have seen people who came from families that invested heavily into their five relationship needs accounts develop horrible decision-making ability.

You are required to accept responsibility for your actions, vice blaming someone else or your environment. Accepting responsibility for your actions is a sign of emotional maturity and stability. Habitual bad decision-making is a symptom of a person in the midst of a personal crisis. People in a crisis require radical, not subtle change to overcome their past, which begins first with making a decision to accept responsibility for your decisions and then submitting yourself to an environment capable of helping you to reform your past behavior. Acknowledging where you are is the first and most important step in the twelve step recovery process.

Actions versus Intentions

Have you ever wanted to fulfill a commitment/obligation and before it was consummated, were asked by the recipient, why it was not done? This is an example of an unmet expectation. In our relationships there will be times when we do not completely fulfill our commitments/obligations. During the conversation with the recipient, both parties may identify some valid reasons for the delay or lack of fulfillment of the commitment/obligation. There may also be times when it is hard to justify why we failed (e.g., false statements of capabilities, laziness or willful disregard of the recipient's needs). A truthful response, which could create further disappointment, is the best response. Unexecuted intentions manifested in our failure to live up to commitments/obligations have the greatest impact on our acceptance and trust relationship needs accounts. Additionally, our intentions (thoughts in our heads unknown by others) can create blind spots in our evaluation of our joint relationship needs accounts. The blind spots could cause us to think the relationship needs accounts are in good standing, when in fact, they are overdrawn. Habitual failure to live up to commitments/obligations will severely damage our reputation and will result in negative relationship needs account balances. Therefore, it is wise to carefully evaluate commitments/obligations and when necessary, clearly communicate to the recipient, a delay or inability to completely fulfill the commitment/obligation. Understanding our capabilities and/or limitations and acknowledging that our actions do speak louder than intentions, can minimize withdrawals and contribute to the growth of assets in our joint relationship needs accounts.

Peers' Impact on Decisions

As I stated in chapter 1, "Love," I said. "I think it is important to address how do you find a group of people worthy of your association ("Remember the path of least resistance" and "Show me your friends and I will show you your future")." Your choice of peers can have a significant impact on your environment and whether or not it is conducive to good decision-making.

During my decades of travel, I have seen the results of a person's peers on their decision-making process. The need to feel accepted is the primary reason why your peers can influence your decision-making. Acceptance can have some disastrous or positive results (remember what Mr. Dale Carnegie said about the books you read and the people you meet!) A friend of mine, used to tell his sons, that if you are the smartest person in your group of friends, it is time to find some new friends! If your peers do not encourage you to practice self-control, self-discipline, or strive to be the best that you can be, you could be heading for trouble. Even if you choose not to involve yourself in the destructive behavior of your peers, it is unrealistic to think you will avoid the consequences of their decisions. Suffering the consequences of your own decisions can be costly, but I think it would be tragic to suffer the consequences from someone else's decisions (e.g. being a passenger in a vehicle with someone who has a chosen to drink and drive or a passenger in a stolen vehicle).

I encourage you to associate with peers who do not use unhealthy coercion to get you to do something you do not want to do. For example, if you are out and choose to limit your drinking to one or two beers over a period of four hours because you know you have to go school or work the next morning, your peers, who are worthy of your acquaintance, will respect your desire to limit your consumption of alcohol. There will be times when you will have to go it alone, and just say "No" regardless of the action the group decides to take. It's better to be the one going to the memorial service, than to be the one being remembered. Either situation is tragic, but walking away could in some cases, be the difference between life and death! Having the moral courage to say "No" can be easier, if you have identified with your own spirituality and establish healthy boundaries.

Language

One of the most powerful tools that is available to you, is language, both aural and written. Your words can etch in the minds of others your character and reflect who you are as a person. Words can either magnify or defile a person. Many a great man and woman were forced to retire or lost authority because of their choice of words. One of the biggest challenges is remembering to think before we speak. We may live in a free society, but that does not excuse us from being held accountable for our use of words.

I grew up in an era when profanity and explicit description of sexual acts were practically banned from radio and television broadcasts and there was no internet to support "underground" distribution. It is now almost passé for profanity, the N-word, which I consider to be a racial slur (CEO's have been relieved for its use) and sexual explicits that are uttered freely with little to no restraints. I am especially appalled at the use of this type of language that is used regularly by young people or entertainers whose music attracts younger listeners. I have heard teenagers spew words of profanity and/or racial slurs that are totally unacceptable, especially when it is spoken to or about persons of authority (remember, respect is reciprocal!) It is a shame that there is not an emphasis on promoting good vocabulary and very little reinforcement in today's media outlets.

I believe there should be a sensitivity about use of language, especially when in the presence of children and elders. Good language usage does not happen by accident (as a retired sailor, I believe I am qualified to make this statement!), and requires constant thinking before speaking. If your peers do not use language that is appropriate, it is easy for you to fall into a pattern of inappropriate language usage. As a sailor, I was in an environment where inappropriate language was almost the accepted norm. It was not until I consciously decided not to use offensive language (the N-word was never part of my vocabulary), that I was able to repeatedly express myself without the fear of offending others. To manage this behavior required and still requires, daily attention and prayer. I believe freedom of expression means we have freedom to use language that is not offensive or oppressive. Freedom does not equal recklessness, but willingly conforming to defined boundaries! Preservation of freedom requires continuous acceptance, that we share the responsibility to use words that reflect respect for the privileges associated with living in a free society.

Clothing

Your clothing communicates just as loudly as your voice. Deciding to intentionally "sag" your pants or to wear clothing that does not properly cover your body, does little to encourage respectful interactions. I once heard a minister state the three "C's" of clothing. He said your clothes "Communicate," "Compliment," and "Cover." In addition to choosing the words that you express, your choice of clothing and / or decision on how to wear your clothes can also have detrimental consequences. There are numerous examples of how an individual's choice in clothing had detrimental impacts on their treatment or perception of their character. Similar to your choice of language, your choice of clothing can either compliment or defile your character. Therefore, your choice of clothing is essential to assisting you in achieving your long-term objectives.

Threat to America's Freedom

When America's founding fathers wrote the Constitution, it was based on the belief that men and women freely choose to exercise their moral conscience. "Domestic tranquility" was one of the basic frameworks for independence from governmental control and domination. America's citizens have an obligation to control their conduct in public and in private and to strive for peaceful cohabitation with their neighbors. Today, the concept of self-discipline is being replaced with "no one caught me" or "it is my right." It is my belief, that if America's citizens continue to ignore the need for individual accountability and responsibility, the "blessings of liberty to ourselves and our posterity" will be lost for its future generations. True freedom begins with knowing you have a choice to either behave morally or amorally. True character is defined as what you do when no one else is around and requires self-discipline, which for most people, preferred over totalitarian governmental control.

Life's Journey, with or without External Stimulates?

The story of the young man who died due to alcohol poisoning is a warning about the use of external stimulants. Had he not been drinking all day prior to his deathly act, he probably would have concluded, that his decision to drink a fifth of a bottle of liquor would cost him his life! When I discussed the relationship needs accounts (love, acceptance, appreciation, respect, and trust) I stated how they can affect your relationships. I want to introduce another concept, which is related to your five relationship needs accounts and that is your desire to remain connected to reality. Some people have strong urges to escape their reality and use external stimulates to assist them on their mind-altering experience. Regardless of how desperate your economic position or the status of your five relationship needs accounts, the use of external stimulants won't resolve any of your problems. I stated earlier, there are numerous examples of people who did not address their relationship needs accounts and suffered tragic consequences such as death due to suicide or drug overdose.

Your family history can provide you some insight on whether or not you are more susceptible than others when it comes to alcohol or drug addiction. Not all people are created equal when it comes to external stimulants. There are some stimulates that cannot be experimented with at all and initial contact can lead to death or addition. Some people may be able to experiment with alcohol, but I strongly discourage all drug use (including experimentation) legal or illegal and if you choose to consume alcohol, that you first take a look at your family history. Because of brain development, I believe that individuals under the age of twenty-six should not experiment with marijuana or any other stimulants! Even for people who do not have a personal family history of alcohol or drug abuse, they need to realize the use of external stimulants will have destructive results. You may have to choose to completely abstain in order to avoid placing yourself in situations where your sense of judgment is severely impaired, for some people that occurs even after one or two drinks of alcohol. Some activities are too dangerous to introduce even mild effects of impairment, such as driving an automobile or using heavy machinery, and as such, most states in America are lowering their blood to alcohol content level from 1.0 to 0.8 for driving under the influence (DUI) convictions.

I once had a friend who had a difficult time managing his use of external stimulants. His habitual use of alcohol and drugs began when he was a teenager and led to a life of hard times. He was eventually gunned downed at the age of thirty-five by a jealous boyfriend of one of his female co-drug users. Unfortunately, he never grew up and lived from one party to the next and then jail time to parties that eventually ended with his untimely death. His death affected all of his family, friends (including me), and especially his three children who were left without a father. Alcohol and drugs severely impair your ability to make good decisions. When you have any combination of overdrawn relationship needs accounts, immoral peers, alcohol or drug abuse, or lack of spiritually aligned moral convictions; you have a lethal environment that will result in destructive consequences.

Putting It All Together

I hope my words have encouraged you to look into your emotional seabag and check the contents. If you have at least identified what is in your seabag and started thinking of ways to check the status of your relationship needs accounts and make necessary adjustments to fill them, then you are on your way to leading a fulfilling life. Life is a continuum of exploring and learning. You have the opportunity to learn from the consequences of your decisions or from the insight gained from others, because hindsight is not always twenty-twenty. Once you have humbled yourself to realize that you still have a lot to learn, you can begin to add to your existing collection of relative knowledge and begin identifying sources of wisdom. I believe an ounce of humility can yield a gallon of knowledge!

I believe that when one emotionally independent and stable man enters into a union with an equally-equipped woman, it has the ability to produce a joy that few other life experiences can compete with. The ability to have a relationship that has the potential to produce children who can carry on a legacy is priceless. To have a relationship of that quality is worth the wait, especially if during the waiting period, you are preparing yourself to achieve success in other areas of your life. The decision on the quality of relationship you will have with your spouse is partially yours and partially your spouse's. Some see marriage, as the "end" instead of the viewing marriage as the "beginning." If you see your decision as the beginning of a new journey, that has the potential for contentment, you are halfway to having the quality you should expect in a lifelong relationship.

There will be times when your sense of determination and faith will be tested. Your sense of determination and faith will be tested during times of personal loss or other tragedies. There is a proverb that says, "If thou faint in the day of adversity, thy strength is small" (Proverbs 24:10). That Proverb has provided me comfort during my times of tribulation and is an unending sense of hope, which is based on my faith in God vice people. My faith in God is reassuring and reminds me that despite how tough things might get, God is able to see me through the situation. No one goes through life without experiencing some losses. The courage to decide to persevere despite a gloomy forecast depends greatly on what is the basis of your faith (God or man?) Without a strong sense of faith, I have seen people who looked like impenetrable towers of strength, crumble like pillars of salt when the wrecking ball of tragedy strikes. Everyone needs something to believe in and without faith during your times of peace and during times of tribulation, it will be difficult to find the courage to decide to "press on."

Understanding the "why" behind your decisions is important if you desire not to repeat past mistakes. Hindsight is only twenty-twenty when you are willing to accept responsibility for your past, along with its bad and good attributes. When it is all said and done, you can either be remembered by what you gave to others or how much you stole from humanity. You should strive to lead a life that is reverent toward the gift of life. You can make a difference; it's up to you to make the decision to get involved and live up to your commitments! The best gift you can provide to society is to leave behind a generation of emotionally healthy children to take your place. The best environment for producing emotionally healthy children is within a marital relationship. If you have resolved your issues prior to marriage, then you stand a good chance of being able to express your Love to your spouse, to your children, family, friends and society.

The One with the Most Toys Wins? Not!

Once you are equipped with the knowledge that you are just a steward of resources, your "things" take on a different value and a whole new meaning. The ability to hold your possessions with an open hand (in other words, willing to give freely or have little remorse if they are destroyed or stolen), demonstrates you have the maturity required to maintain them and pass them on to future generations. The ability to acquire wealth depends on how many seeds you planted in your life. If you planted good seeds in soil that is rich in resources, then you can expect a bountiful harvest. Let me make it clear that wealth is not just monetary! Wealth is a healthy family, lifelong friends, emotionally-stable children, contributions to society, spiritual salvation, and many more rewards that money can't buy! In order to have plants worthy of harvesting, you have to plant early and with discipline and faith. You also have to have the self-discipline to deny yourself of some luxuries today in hopes of higher future returns.

Having a balanced life requires many adjustments along life's precarious road. You have to make deposits and limited withdrawals to the five relationship needs accounts in your relationships, make adjustments based on reassessments, value your relationships, and focus on a moral vision fueled by faith.

Calvin Coolidge, a former US president (1923–1929), is noted for saying "Nothing in the world can take the place of persistence. Talent will not; nothing is more common than unsuccessful men of talent. Genius will not; the world is full of educated derelicts. Persistence and determination alone are omnipotent. The slogan 'press on' has solved, and will always solve, the problems of the human race."

If you don't have that undying persistence to continue or "press on" when times are tough, you will never achieve personal success.

That means doing things that may at times seem unpleasant and/or require personal sacrifice. The ability to make sacrifices in order to do what is morally right is a sign of being at peace with yourself and reflects strength of character.

Your word has value. A person is respected when they say what they mean and mean what they say. A person who is respected will be far more spiritually wealthy, than someone who cheated their way to the top. When a person is known for being trustworthy, their word is more precious than the finest jewels. Your word and reputation are truly priceless and are essential ingredients to maintaining healthy relationships.

I would like to share with you a quote by an anonymous writer. These words should remind you that your decisions are important to your destiny. Your first decision is to decide what you allow to occupy your thoughts. What you meditate on is what you become; therefore, you become what you think.

Character Is Destiny

> Be careful of your thoughts,
> For your thoughts become your words;
> Be careful of your words,
> For your words become your deeds;
> Be careful of your deeds,
> For your deeds become your habits;

CLEVELAND O. EASON

> Be careful of your habits,
> For your habits become your character;
> Be careful of your character,
> For your character becomes your destiny.

In this day and age, when people seemingly make their choices with little regard to the consequences, it is important for you to have a firm set of principles to live by. Being at peace with yourself, your family, friends, and neighbors (balanced relationship needs accounts) allows you to be an asset vice liability to your community. Regardless of your religious preference, I hope you can apply the following principles, which is an adaptation from Saint Francis of Assisi's prayer into your daily life. When you seek to understand more than to be understood, love more than to be loved, forgive more than to be forgiven, serve rather than to be served, then you are on your way to realizing a journey that will be consummated in a strong finish in life's marathon. I hope that your life will be filled with memories of how much you gave to edify the lives of others and savor the rewards of being a good steward. Remember, it is better to give than to receive and if we love our neighbor as we love ourselves, then the world becomes a better place for present and future generations.

In closing, I'd like to remind you of one the reasons for this book. I wrote this book because I believe if you are willing to learn from my collage of experiences and limit learning from the School of Hard Knocks, then your life's journey has the potential to be harmonious and profitable. Good luck (in other words, have a vision, work hard, and be persistent!), and I challenge you to cherish each day, for the time we spend on this earth is nonrefundable and truly priceless!